Henrik Vejlgaard

LOOK YOUNGER WITHOUT SURGERY

LEARN TO RADIATE YOUTHFULNESS

CONFETTI PUBLISHING

ISBN-10: 193923543X
ISBN-13: 978-1-939235-43-5

Library of Congress Control Number: 2012917854

Published by Confetti Publishing

www.confettipublishing.com

IMPORTANT NOTICE/DISCLAIMER
The contents of this book are intended to be entertaining in the
tradition of magazine articles and are NOT intended and should
NOT be relied upon as recommending or promoting a specific
method, diagnosis, or treatment by physicians or other health
professionals. The publisher and author specifically disclaim
any liability, loss or risk, personal or otherwise, which is in-
curred as a consequence, directly or indirectly, of the use and
application of any of the contents of this book.

CONTENTS

INTRODUCTION

Understanding How to Look Younger

Page 9

If you feel younger than you look, now you have a chance to look the age you feel.

CHAPTER 1

Finding Your True Age

Page 13

By thinking not only of your biological age but also your self-perceived age, you can start working on your visual age—the age you want to convey to other people.

CHAPTER 2

How Not to Reveal Your Age

Page 20

If you want to change people's perceptions of your age, you have to understand what reveals your age and start changing the signs that give your age away.

CHAPTER 3

Looking at the Body

Page 27

Our body is a big giveaway of our age—with or without clothes. It's all about weight, height, posture, breasts, and skin.

CHAPTER 4

Test Your Fashion Profile

Page 45

The most important step in looking younger is to rethink what you wear. Find out if your current style is sending the right youthful signals.

CHAPTER 5

Dress Your Desired Visual Age

Page 53

By following these style guidelines, you can be sure that your style matches your desired visual age.

CHAPTER 6

Flaunting Your Youthful Image

Page 57

Accessories are powerful age signifiers. Though they are only a small part of what you wear, their effect is greater than their size.

CHAPTER 7

Facing Your Face

Page 63

There are several things that can be done in order to continue having or getting a youthful face. It's all about skin and teeth.

CHAPTER 8

Visionary Cues

Page 84

Eyewear can effectively be used to cue people you meet into your desired visual age.

CHAPTER 9

Young-Looking Hair Days

Page 93

Knowing exactly how your hair reveals your age to other people makes it easy to do something about these signals.

CHAPTER 10

Using Make-up the Youthful Way

Page 101

By following make-up trends, you can disguise your biological age and look younger.

CHAPTER 11

Moving Signals

Page 110

How you care for your hands and feet will give the final touches to a more youthful you.

CHAPTER 12

Fragrances for Any Age

Page 114

Trends in fragrance can be used to highlight the signals we are sending with our clothes, accessories, hair, and make-up.

CHAPTER 13

Lifestyle Accessories

Page 117

There are many lifestyle products that send youthful signals. The most important lifestyle accessories are cell phones, music players, laptops, and luggage.

CHAPTER 14

Cues for the Young Mind

Page 120

Make sure that you share interests and conversation not only with people your own age but also with people whose biological age matches your self-perceived age.

CHAPTER 15

Getting Started

Page 131

Now that you have an over-view of how to look more like the age you feel, it is time to get started looking younger.

Understanding How to Look Younger

You are not the only one who wants to look younger. Millions of women and men feel the same way. All have very good reasons for this: They *feel* younger than they look. Now you have the chance to look the age *you* feel. With this book, you will get inspiration and guidance on all the options that are available to you if you want to look younger.

There are many ways to start looking younger. Some of these options you may be aware of, but with this book, you will not only get a complete overview of all options but also inspiration and guidance on how to make the best of them.

When we want to look younger, we have to be aware of the many signals or clues that give away our age. In particular, what we wear gives away our age. This book is about using these signals and clues to give a youthful impression to the world. Many will be surprised by how much younger they can look by just changing a few of these signals and clues.

The book is not about getting to look a certain age. It is a book that recognizes that people are different and have different needs and different attitudes towards their age. In order to help you in the best way possible, you must start by taking the Self-Perceived Age Quiz in the next chapter. The quiz helps you establish your desired visual age.

TOOLS AND GUIDELINES

When you know your desired visual age, you can start using the tools and guidelines in the book. The tools and guidelines have been created to help you no matter your biological age. But if your biological age is between forty and seventy years, you will probably stand to benefit the most from this book.

The Self-Perceived Age Quiz and the other tests and tools in this book are unique. You will not have encountered the tests and tools in other books or magazines.

When you use it, you will realize that the book is like having your own personal style consultant at your disposal. But this style consultant not only guides you on how to look good, but more importantly, also how to look *younger*. We can look good at any age, but looking younger takes a whole different approach than just looking good. It takes an in-depth knowledge of the mechanisms that determine what youthfulness is.

SURGERY NOT REQUIRED

Cosmetic surgery is often thought of as one of the most effective ways of looking younger. Whether you have had cosmetic surgery or not—or will in the future—you will be able to benefit from this book. However, the focus of the book is to guide and inspire you in what you yourself can do to look the age you feel, both what can be done actively to look younger and what can be done to prevent some of the signs of aging. The book does *not* give advice on cosmetic surgery, but there are brief overviews of some medical and dental options available to people who want to look younger.

Look Younger Without Surgery is full of easy-to-use instructions. Please be aware that the book is focused on looking younger. It is *not* a book about the basics of general skincare, beauty, or health. Therefore, you will *not* find advice on, for instance, removing facial and body hair, general hair care, or how to apply make-up.

You can read the entire book, or you can just pick and choose the information that you feel you need most right now; at other times, you may want to read other parts. The content is structured so that if you are looking for specific information, it is easy to get an overview of each chapter right from the start of the chapter.

What Kind of Research
Is the Book Based on?

The tests, tools, and guides in this book are based on the research and thinking of three books, all by the author of *Look Younger Without Surgery*. These are *Anatomy of a Trend*, which is about trends and trendsetters; *The Lifestyle Puzzle*, which is about the signals that our clothes and accessories tell other people about us; and *Style Eruptions*, which is about how changes in style take place. All three books are based on meticulous observation of thousands of women and men of different ages.

Specifically, this book is based on three different kinds of research:

❖ Studies of what constitutes what is young and youthful in our society.

❖ An understanding of how style changes and insight into trends that affect many people.

❖ Research on all the different things you can do to look younger.

Finding Your True Age

CHAPTER FOCUS
❖ Biological age
❖ Self-perceived age
❖ Desired visual age

You know how old you are according to your birth certificate, but how *young* do you feel? Before you can start using the information and tools in this book, take some time to determine what age you want to convey to other people. This may be somewhere between your biological age and the age you feel you are. By thinking not only of our biological age but also our self-perceived age, we can meaningfully start working on our visual age—the age we want to convey to the people we meet. Now it is time to find the age you want to look!

Age is no longer just about our biological age, as determined by the date on our birth certificate. Today many people feel that they are younger than the age that their birth certificate says they are. For some, it is just a few years; for others, it can be several decades. No matter how many years, it is only natural that we want to *look* the age we feel.

Feeling young, dressing young, and acting young is not limited to a certain age. There are no rules anymore that say you can only do certain things at a certain age. No matter what your age is, as long as you are fit, you can go roller-skating, scuba-diving, and travel around the world.

We all feel and see that our bodies and faces change as we grow older. Sixty percent of general aging is due to genetics, which we can do little—or nothing—about. The remaining forty percent depends on how we live our lives. For example, work, stress, worries, sun bathing, and smoking influence how we look. This also means that we have some influence on a rather big part of the aging process.

We are not as limited by our biological age as we were in past centuries. These days, many people have jobs that do not require hard physical labor. This means that wear and tear on the body is different for many people as compared to fifty years ago. The result is that we often do not look or feel our biological age.

Age Elasticity

We have introduced the term *age elasticity* for the phenomenon in which you see yourself as younger than your biological age. Age elasticity is the difference between

❖ Biological age: the age according to your birth certificate.

❖ Self-perceived age: the age at which you perceive yourself.

Today, a person's self-perceived age is most likely younger than his or her biological age. A person's biological age may be forty-five years, but her self-perceived age could be thirty-five—or even younger.

You do not have to have a certain age elasticity to use the information in this book, but the higher your age elasticity, the more you can probably gain from the book's tools.

Age elasticity applies to both women and men. But, generally, men's age elasticity is higher than women's. It is not uncommon for men in their fifties to see themselves as being twenty-five years old. There are different reasons for men's higher age elasticity; the main reason probably is that men can father children for more years than women can give birth to children (at least the natural way).

HOW MEN FEEL ABOUT AGE

For both sexes, it can be disturbing to look in the mirror and see an "old" person when you feel so young inside. This, of course, we want to correct so that we look the age we feel. Men's high age elasticity also makes them sensitive to how their wives and girlfriends look. If a husband and wife are both fifty years old, but the husband feels like a twenty-five-year-old and sees a fifty-year-old woman when he looks at his wife, he may feel there is an imbalance. Though he may himself look like a fifty-year-old, he may be attracted to someone who is closer to his self-perceived age. This explains why, after a divorce, a man may end up with a woman who is younger than his first wife is and younger than himself. (For some women, this is just an extra good reason to get to look the age they feel.)

Find Your Self-perceived Age

If your biological age is between thirty and seventy years, you can take the Self-Perceived Age Quiz to get an indicator of your perceived age. The test will reveal if your perceived age is younger or older than your biological age.

Self-Perceived Age Quiz

Your Biological Age (state your age)	__ Years
If you mostly associate with people who are younger than you, deduct	- 2
If you think you look younger than your biological age, deduct	- 3
If you mostly associate with people who are older than you, add	+ 3
If you truly enjoy experiencing change in your life, deduct	- 3
If you have two or more friends who are more than 10 years younger than you, deduct	- 2
If you live in a city with more than one million inhabitants, deduct	- 1
If you consider yourself conservative in most respects, add	+ 3
If you are curious about what is new in design and style, deduct	- 3
If you buy new, fashionable clothes at least every six months, deduct	-4
If you embrace most new technological developments, deduct	- 2
If you enjoy vacationing in big cities, deduct	- 1
If you are open-minded about how teenagers live their lives, deduct	- 3
If you have not changed your style of dress in the past 10 years, add	+ 3
If you have the same opinions that you did when you were in your 20s, add	+ 2
If you think that everything was much better "in the good old days," add	+ 5
Your approximate self-perceived age	

You know your biological age, and now that you also have an indication of your self-perceived age, you can use this to calculate the age that you want to convey to the world, that is, what you want your visual age to be. The first step in establishing your desired visual age is calculating your suggested visual age. This can be done using the Visual Age Calculator.

Visual Age Calculator

To find your suggested visual age, add your biological age to your self-perceived age and divide by two.

You can choose to convey your self-perceived age or suggested visual age, but if you have a very high age elasticity, you may feel more comfortable with choosing your desired visual age, which is your own modification of your suggested visual age.

EXAMPLE 1

Elizabeth
- ❖ Biological age: 50
- ❖ Self-perceived age: 30
- ❖ Suggested visual age: 40
- ❖ Desired visual age: 40

EXAMPLE 2

Monica
- ❖ Biological age: 61
- ❖ Self-perceived age: 39
- ❖ Suggested visual age: 50
- ❖ Desired visual age: 40

When determining your self-perceived age, you can use the Self-Perceived Age Quiz as inspiration, but you may have a strong feeling yourself of what your self-perceived age is, and this is the number you should use as your self-perceived age in the calculation:

My biological age: _____

My self-perceived age: _____

Suggested visual age: _____

My desired visual age: _____

TALKING ABOUT YOUR AGE

Now that you have a precise idea what age you would like to look, you can start working on your visual age. This is what the rest of this book will help you to do.

But before you start changing your look and style, you should also be aware of how you talk about your age.

If you don't want people to know your biological age and want them to think that you are younger than you are, it does not make sense to tell them your biological age. You should consider avoiding talking about your biological age unless absolutely forced to.

This is not about *not* celebrating your birthdays, and it is not about lying. But when asked about your age, it is perfectly all right to indicate your self-perceived age, not your biological age. If people do not ask for specifics, then *you* choose what age you want to talk about. If you look more like your self-perceived age than your biological age, it actually makes more sense to talk about your self-perceived age.

If asked directly about your age, you can say, "I can tell you my self-perceived age…" or "Age is not in the skin but in the mind—and my mind is only *xx* years old" or "I have stopped talking about my age because age is such a relative concept."

Sometimes, we inadvertently reveal our age by stating the number of years we have been doing this or living there, such as, "I have lived in this apartment for thirty years." If you are around sixty years old, you can give the same information by saying, "I have lived half my life in this apartment." In this way, you can avoid talking about numbers.

Not all people may be aware of the different concepts of age—but more and more people are becoming aware of age elasticity because they feel it themselves.

On your way to looking younger

❖ Acknowledge your self-perceived age.

❖ Choose a visual age between your biological age and your self-perceived age to look convincingly youthful.

❖ Avoid talking about your biological age.

2

How Not to Reveal Your Age

CHAPTER FOCUS
❖ Guessing a person's age
❖ Different approaches to looking younger
❖ Options overview

When you have determined your desired visual age, you want to start changing other people's perceptions of your age. First, you have to know the signals that reveal your age. Then you have to learn how to take advantage of them. It's about using visual signifiers to signal our desired age, but also about reversing and disguising your biological age and sometimes even preventing the changes. There are many options in dealing with age-revealing signals. Luckily, we are in complete control of most of them.

Many women who live in the public eye know the importance of looking younger, and some are very good at looking (much) younger than their biological age. They can be actors, singers, or television personalities. Often we know the biological age of these women (which can make it difficult to be objective about guessing their age), but most people would say that they look younger than their biological age.

Like these women, you can also learn to look younger no matter your biological age. And you will have one advantage over them: People that you meet in public will not know your actual biological age, so it will be easier for you to convey your desired visual age.

The first step in changing people's perceptions of your age is to understand exactly what it is that reveals our age. Both our face and our body are affected by biological changes as we grow older. For most people, these changes first become visible in the face. Often the changes in the body are felt and become visible to others a decade or two later than those affecting the face. The slower visual aging process of the body is a great opportunity for us. It means that we can draw attention to the body—and away from the face—without drawing attention to yet another age revealer. We can use the body to help us signal that we are younger than we are.

We also have to be aware of the many style signals that can reveal our age and sometimes reveal much more than our body. For different reasons, many people do not pay as much attention to the style signals as they do to the body's signals, and consequently, they may end up missing some options that can take years off their age.

We have psychology to help us understand the possibilities the body gives us when we want to look younger. Experts in body language have studied how we look at other human beings when we meet them. Whether we are meeting people for the first time or meeting someone we know well, we use the "vertical scanning approach." When you meet someone, you normally do not just look in the person's eyes. You also look at the person's face and body. Both women and men use the vertical scanning approach, but women use it much more conspicuously than men do.

The Vertical Scanning Approach

When we meet someone, and we want to have a closer look at that person—for whatever reason—we typically start by looking in their eyes. Then we divert our eyes to the upper torso, and then back to the eyes.

Then we divert our eyes again, and this time we may look at the person's hands before looking back to the eyes or face.

Then we look at the hair and then the eyes again.

When we are observing someone or talking to someone for a longer time, we will take in more and more of the body.

Many women also look at the feet of another woman and look at the shoes she is wearing.

There are many different reasons why we use the vertical scanning approach. Some people are shy or don't want to be thought of as flirting. Many people are also naturally curious about what the person is wearing. So they observe. In some cases, their look will be admiring; in other cases, it's the opposite. There are undoubtedly many other reasons why we don't just look at the face of the person we are talking to or of a stranger we are meeting for the first time. But in all instances, we use the vertical scanning approach.

This non-verbal interaction is so very common that we hardly think about it. But it reveals how important what we wear can be to other people's perceptions of us; we can use this to control our image.

The vertical scanning approach is a great opportunity in the quest to look younger because, in this way, we can cue people as to our age using many different clues, not just the skin of our face. Especially from a distance, the body plays a bigger role, not only because it is larger than our face, but also because what we wear is full of clues that other people decode and use to start forming an opinion before we are face to face.

AGE PERCEPTIONS

Imagine you see a woman in the distance. She appears to be forty years old. You guess her age based on the way she dresses, her hairstyle, and the way she moves. From psychology, we know that first impressions count—and that it is in the human mind to want our first impressions, consciously or unconsciously, confirmed. As the woman gets closer, you will automatically want to confirm that she is a forty-year-old woman.

If, in fact, her biological age is fifty, you may think, "Well, for a forty-year-old, she looks her age." You may also adjust your thinking and say to yourself, "Maybe she is forty-five years old." The point is that the way she dresses and the way she moves have made her look younger in your mind, and will probably have done the same in many other people's minds.

On the other hand, if the woman approaching you is only thirty years old, you will think, "Why does she dress older than she is?" or perhaps, "Wow, she looks fantastic for someone who is forty." Again, the message is that our clothes, our hairstyle, make-up, and other visual signals hold strong clues for other people about our age.

This is something that we can take advantage of when we want to convey how old—or rather, how young—we want to look.
The first step is about being aware of the different types of age-revealers and learning how to approach them. You can see different types of age-revealers in the Age-specific Age-revealers Chart.

Age-specific Age-revealers Chart

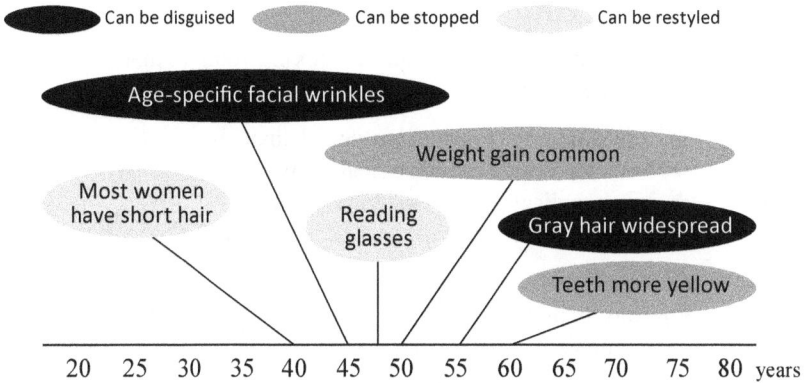

Can be disguised   Can be stopped   Can be restyled

Age-specific facial wrinkles

Weight gain common

Most women
have short hair

Reading
glasses

Gray hair widespread

Teeth more yellow

20 25 30 35 40 45 50 55 60 65 70 75 80 years

Options Overview

Theme	Chapter
Accessories	6
Arms	3
Body	3
Breasts	3
Clothes	5
Eyes	8
Feet	11
Hair	9
Hands	11
Lifestyle	13
Make-up	10
Mentality	14
Posture	3
Teeth	7
Weight	3

4 Different Approaches to Looking Younger

There are different approaches to looking younger that you will learn about in this book:

- ❖ You can prevent (some) biological changes.
- ❖ You can reverse the biological changes.
- ❖ You can disguise the biological changes.
- ❖ You can use visual signifiers to look youthful.

Prevent the biological changes
Preventing biological changes in our body is not easy, but having healthy eating habits and doing sensible exercise on a regular basis can get us a long way.

Reverse the biological changes
Knowing what causes aging gives us a chance—in some cases—to do something about visual aging. We *can* prevent some of the aging of our skin and of our body. For instance, weight gain can be stopped or reversed. We can also do something about the yellowing of teeth.

Disguise the biological changes
Wrinkles and gray hair are two very typical biological age revealers that can be disguised. For instance, in the case of gray hair, this can easily be disguised by coloring the hair. In the case of age-specific face wrinkles, they, too, can be disguised (e.g., with correctly sized *and* trendy eyewear frames).

Use visual signifiers to look youthful
We use visual signifiers to convey our age and deflect attention from the biological changes. Clothing, hairstyles, eyewear, and make-up are typical visual signifiers, but there are many others that you will be introduced to in this book. For instance, we do not have to use reading glasses when we need eyesight correction. There are other options. And for hair length, we can decide the length of our hair ourselves.

On your way to looking younger

❖ Be sure to get an overview of all your options and then choose what will work for you.

❖ Be aware of the age revealers that you yourself can do something about.

❖ Use the visual signifiers that will make you look younger.

3

Looking at the Body

CHAPTER FOCUS
❖ Weight
❖ Height
❖ Posture
❖ Breasts
❖ Skin

When they want to look younger, many people focus on the face and underestimate what the body reveals about their age. But just as most people know what a young face looks like, they also know what a young body looks like. In everyday life, we notice that young people are slimmer and have better posture than old people do. In other words, the body is one big giveaway of our age—with or without clothes. In this chapter, we will look at the body without clothes, so to speak. And in the following three chapters, we will look at the body with clothes.

We learn to interpret certain signs about the body from personal experience, from watching people, and from what we learn from medical science and through the media. Therefore, when we look at a person's body, there are several signs that reveal to us the person's age.

Again and again, we can observe that people put on weight as they grow older. Statistics confirm this, and science explains that one reason for this is that our metabolism changes as we grow older. Therefore, most of us are aware that young people—in general—tend to be slimmer than older people.

Statistics also document that each new generation born since World War II has been taller than the previous one. Today, the average young woman is taller than her mother and her grandmother. Therefore, many people are aware that young women tend to be taller than older women.

Sports and exercise are something that we mostly see young people do, and we notice that there are fewer old people doing sports and exercise. This also helps confirm that young women tend to have fitter bodies than older women.

BODY LANGUAGE

As we grow old, our body language changes. We become more hesitant, we have less flexible bodies, and we are less agile.

The bone structure of our bodies starts changing when we reach a certain age. For women, especially, the bone structure is affected by the hormonal changes that are connected to menopause. There may be other reasons why a woman slouches more as she ages. The point is that many people know that young women tend to stand more erect than older women do.

Women's breast sizes vary greatly. The size can change when aging (for many different reasons) and so can the shape. But no matter the size, most people know that young women tend to have firmer breasts than older women do.

SIGNS OF AGING

The skin on our faces changes, and so does the skin on our bodies. With age, the skin on the body becomes wrinkled, liver spots develop, and cellulite may also show up on many parts of the body. Again, we are well aware that younger women tend to have smoother skin than older women do.

So, we know what makes us look older in the eyes of the world (and in our own eyes as well). On the other hand, we also know what can make us look younger:

- ❖ If you are slim, you are younger looking.
- ❖ If you are tall, you are younger looking .
- ❖ If you are fit, you are younger looking.
- ❖ If you are agile, you are younger looking.
- ❖ If you have a good posture, you are younger looking.
- ❖ If you have firm breasts, you are younger looking.
- ❖ If you have smooth skin, you are younger looking.

The first step in changing people's perceptions of our age is considering these facts. If something can be done on one or more of these aspects of the body, it can help you look younger.

Let us take a closer look at each element and see what can be prevented, what can be reversed, and what can be disguised. There are, inevitably, things that you cannot do anything about. Don't be frustrated by this because there are so many other things that you can do something about.

WEIGHT ISSUES

Most people gain weight as they grow older, often because our metabolism changes. If we keep eating the same number of calories as we grow older that we ate when we were young, we will eventually gain weight. There are also other reasons people gain weight, and there are many good reasons to avoid it. Health is one of them, but it is also about looking youthful.

Habit Changing Weight Control Program

If you want to prevent weight gain, avoid gaining *more* weight, or lose weight you have gained as an adult, you should adopt the *Look Younger Magazine* Weight Control Program. This program is not about a certain diet. It is about changing habits.

Shopping habits

❖ Buy food that is high in protein. One gram of protein contains only four calories per gram. One gram of carbohydrates also contains four calories. Though proteins and carbohydrates contain the same number of calories it is better to get more protein than carbohydrates for two reasons. 1) You will stay fuller for a longer period of time when eating protein. 2) Calories from carbohydrates may come from sugar and other fast carbohydrates, of which we do not need a lot. Too much sugar is stored as fat. One gram of fat contains nine calories, and one gram of alcohol contains seven calories. If you eat 100 grams of protein and feel full, you have consumed only 400 calories. If you eat 100 grams of fat and then feel full, you will have consumed 900 calories. In both cases you feel full, but you will have gained less weight by eating proteins.

❖ In general, avoid buying packaged food that does not have a nutrition facts label. With a nutrition facts label, you can learn how much fat, carbohydrates, or protein you will be eating.

❖ In general, avoid buying food that contains a lot of fat. On average, a maximum of 30% of the number of calories in the food you buy should come from fat.

❖ Be critical when buying "light" or "diet" products. Some light or diet products contain lots of sugar. If you eat more sugar than your body can use, you will gain weight.

Eating habits

❖ Avoid fatty and oily foods whenever possible; that is, when you have an option to choose something else, do so.

❖ Avoid butter, margarine, mayonnaise, and similar fatty foods whenever you can; that is, when the food has not already been prepared.

- ❖ Avoid sugar as much as possible. That is, avoid soft drinks, candy, and other sugary drinks and food. If you want to snack, eat fruit or vegetables instead.
- ❖ Eat fibers often, and especially in the morning. This will keep you full longer.
- ❖ Avoid fast food, not only because it is generally more fattening than regular food but also because we eat fast food quickly with the risk of overeating.
- ❖ Avoid low-calorie soft drinks. They can trick your body and brain into feeling hungry. Drink water and/or skim milk instead. Sometimes you can drink fruit or vegetable juices as an alternative.
- ❖ If you use food to comfort yourself, prepare food with as few calories as possible.
- ❖ Don't avoid foods that you really like even if the food is "bad" for you. However, try to eat it at special occasions, for instance, when you are celebrating.
- ❖ Even if you eat healthy food, you should never eat any more food than what it takes to make you feel full. Even healthy food contains calories that will make you gain weight.
- ❖ Avoid snacking between breakfast and lunch. Often, snacking between breakfast and lunch is more about habits than about being hungry.
- ❖ It is better to eat several small meals than a few big meals—as long as you don't take in more calories when you eat those small meals. In this way, you will not get to feel so hungry that you eat more than you need.

Mealtime habits

- ❖ Eat slowly—actually eat as slowly as possible. It takes about 20 minutes for your brain to register that your stomach is full. When your brain has registered that you have food in your stomach, the hunger will go away.
- ❖ Stop eating before you feel full. If your stomach is full after 10 minutes of eating, it will be about 20 minutes before your brain will tell you to stop eating. This means that you can go on eating food that you don't really need. The slower you eat, the less risk of overeating.

- Only eat when you are hungry, but try to avoid waiting to eat till you are very hungry because you are then more likely to eat more before your brain registers that you are full.
- Never bring all the food to the table, whether you're eating out of pans or off of plates. When not socializing, leave some food in the kitchen.
- Separate food from entertainment. We eat faster when we watch television because we don't talk, and because we eat faster we will end up eating more than we need.
- Avoid using big plates for dinner. It will make you put more food on the plate. Use small ones instead.
- Eat with a small fork and/or small spoon. This will make you eat more slowly.
- Be conscious about taking a second helping—don't make it a routine to have seconds.
- Eat meals that consist of a maximum of two courses when not socializing.
- In every twenty-four-hour period, make sure that there are at least eight hours during which you do not eat. For most people, this means not eating during the night.

CHANGE YOUR HABITS PERMANENTLY

If you need to make major adjustments in your diet in order to stop gaining weight or to lose weight, change one or two habits at a time. To change all your habits at once can be hard. For many people, it will be more effective in the long run to stop one weight-gaining habit every two weeks or every month. Shopping habits should be changed right away.

If you follow the basic anti-weight gaining information above, it does not matter what specific kind of diet you choose, if any. The important thing is that you eat and drink fewer calories than you burn.

If you want to be successful in achieving your weight goals, it is important to change your habits permanently, not just temporarily. But be sure to change them in a way you can sustain for a long time. If you are really unhappy with what you eat, there is a greater risk of getting back to habits that will make you gain weight.

LOOKING TALL

The statistics speak loud and clear: Young people are taller than the previous generation. When comparing women in a young age group and a mid-life age group, we can see that there is more than a one-inch difference in the typical height between women in their thirties and women in their sixties.

Models and Miss America contestants are taller than these averages. In the United States and in Europe, top models are ideally 5 ft 11 to 6 ft tall (178–180 cm).

As men also are getting taller, the traditional difference in height between men and women continues to exist.

Age Group	Median Height*
30s	5 ft 4 (163 cm)**
60s	5 ft 3 (160 cm)**

When we reach our late teens, we stop growing, and this is the height we remain for most of our lives. Some people will lose height, some because of bad posture and some because of hormonal and other changes in their body.

We cannot change our height when we are grown up, but we *can* prevent bad posture (more on this later in this chapter), and women can use heels to help them look taller.

To look younger by wearing heels, you can use the Height and Heels Coordinating Guidelines.

---

* This measure divides the age distribution into two equal parts: one-half of the population falling below the median value and one-half above the median value.

** Numbers relate to Caucasian women, the tallest group

Height and Heels Coordinating Guidelines

Height	Heels
Under 5 ft 3 (160 cm)	Aim for 2½-inch (6 cm) heels or higher, as long as you are comfortable
5 ft 3 – 5 ft 4½ (160 – 164 cm)	Aim for at least 2½-inch (6 cm) heels
5 ft 5 – 5 ft 6 (165 – 170 cm)	Aim for at least 2-inch (5 cm) heels
5 ft 6½ – 5 ft 8½ (171 – 176 cm)	Aim for at least 1½-inch heels (4 cm) heels
Over 5 ft 8½ (over 176 cm)	Aim for 1-inch (2½ cm) heels or what makes you comfortable

You cannot wear shoes with heels all the time, of course, but use shoes with heels as much as possible, as long as the shoes, sandals, boots, etc. also signal youthfulness (more on this in the following chapters, specifically Chapter Six, on accessories).

THE FIT BODY

Depending on where you live and where you go on vacation, you will probably be wearing clothing that will show some skin—maybe a t-shirt or a sleeveless dress. This is when you also reveal how fit your body is and something about your biological age. There is no doubt that a fit body is younger-looking than a non-fit body.

If you want to change the looseness of your skin and the contours of your body, exercise is an important activity. There are many ways to stay fit, and it does not matter what kind of exercise you choose, as long as it achieves what you want to achieve and you are motivated to do it regularly. It is better to do a little exercise that you really like than something that you will try to skip. If you want to work on the looseness of your skin and the contours of your body, you can get inspiration from the Fit Body Activity Guide.

The Fit Body Activity Guide

Activity		Firmer Skin	Muscle Definition
	Weight control program	X	
	Walking/race walking	X	Lower body
	Jogging	X	Lower body
	Bicycling	X	Lower body
	Aerobic exercise	X	X
	Stair-climbing machine	X	Lower body
	Swimming	X	X
	Rowing (also in machine)	X	X
	Training with weights or machines	X	X

Worth Knowing: Liposuction

If you want to have a fit-looking body and don't have the time or patience to go through weight control and/or exercise, liposuction may be an alternative. Liposuction is the removal of fat cells by surgery. Liposuction is mostly used to remove fat deposits from the hips, stomach, and thighs, but can be done in many areas of the body and the chin. The surgical procedure removes the fat and reduces the number of fat cells in the area so that fat will not come back so easily in this area. Liposuction should be performed by an experienced plastic surgeon.

There are many reasons to focus on doing exercises—sports and exercise can be fun, your health improves, and you get a young-looking body. There are also many reasons why people do not keep fit: lack of time, lack of energy, and lack of knowledge are some of them.

If your aim is to have a fit body in order to look younger—and you have reasons for not doing any kind of full-body exercise—you can get away with less: just focus on the arms. While focusing on the arms will not improve your overall health, it can help you look younger. The arms are important because they are the part of the body that is most likely to be visible to other people when you wear a T-shirt, a short-sleeved dress, or a sleeveless dress.

The upper arms are the big age revealer of the upper body. The upper arm consists of two muscles: biceps and triceps. If these two muscles are firm, this can help signal a youthful, firm body.

It is never too late to start working on the muscles of the upper arm. At almost any age, they can get firmer. So if you cannot do any other kind of exercise, the Basic Biceps and Triceps Exercise Program will help you have firm upper arms. The exercises can be done almost anywhere at any time.

Basic Biceps and Triceps Exercise Program

The exercises should be done every second day when starting the program. After three months, the program can be continued two to three times a week, depending on how toned you want the arms be. Warm up by swinging your arms back and forth twenty-five times, both to the sides and up in the air.

Biceps Exercise

Arm bending with dumbbells

1. Sit down on a chair without armrests with your legs wider apart than the shoulders.
2. Place your left hand on your upper left leg for support.
3. Place the right elbow on the upper right leg for support.
4. Let your right arm hang down with the dumbbell in your right hand.
5. Raise your right arm to your chest while getting elbow support from the upper leg.
6. Lower the right arm to starting position.

Do ten repetitions with right arm, then ten repetitions with the left arm. Do this three times in all.

Triceps Exercise

Push-ups on knees

1. Lay down on the floor on your stomach.
2. Lift your feet off the floor, but keep your knees on the floor.
3. Cross your ankles.
4. Place your hands on the floor underneath your shoulders.
5. Raise your arms so that you lift your upper body.
6. Keep the body straight while lowering the arms.
7. Be careful not to lock your elbows when arms are stretched.

Do one set of eight to ten repetitions.

It is best to use dumbbells when doing the exercises. If you have not done any biceps or triceps training before, you should probably only start with two-pound dumbbells and then use heavier weights as you get stronger. Always stop exercising if you feel any kind of discomfort.

If you do not have dumbbells, you can use a book, a big bottle of shampoo, a candlestick, or any other object that is easy to hold and has the right weight for you.

BEING MORE FLEXIBLE

When we grow older, our body language also changes. We move more slowly and our movements become more hesitant. Generally, this has to do with the body becoming less flexible. When this happens, we often become more careful with physical activities. While being careful is always wise, it is also wise to work on keeping the body as agile as possible. Being flexible will make you feel better and look younger.

The good news is that inflexibility can be reversed. In one study on how to improve flexibility, two groups of men were compared to each other. One group was comprised of teenagers and the other of seniors (aged 63 to 88). The study documented that both groups could become more flexible with equal ease.

The best way to stay flexible and agile is doing sports and exercise. If that is not an option, the Dynamic Movement Exercise Program is a good alternative. Dynamic movement consists of many different exercises that will make you stay flexible and improve coordination.

Dynamic Movement Exercise Program

The exercises should be done twice a week. Warm up by hopping up and down twenty-five times.

Rolling Down

1. Stand upright with feet placed wider than the shoulders.
2. Raise your arms out to the sides, a little higher than horizontal position.
3. Relax your knees.
4. Slowly bend your head and arms towards the floor.
5. Slowly continue rolling your head towards the floor, letting the arms move to the floor first.
6. Try to let the fingers touch the floor (bend the knees if necessary).
7. Roll slowly up to starting position.

Repeat exercise three times.

Sitting Cross Reach

1. Sit down on the floor with your back straight, legs straight in front of you.
2. Place your left arm behind your back as support, legs straight in front of you.
3. Raise your right arm and slowly move it towards your left foot.
4. Bring back right arm and use it as support behind your back.
5. Raise your left arm and slowly move it towards your right foot.

Repeat ten times.

Standing Diagonal Reach

1. Stand up with feet apart.
2. Bend the right leg while the left leg is stretched out to the side.
3. Place the right hand on the right knee.
4. Place the left hand in front of the lower right leg.
5. Slowly bring the left arm across your chest and up in the air.
6. Bring left arm back to starting position.

Repeat five times with left arm, then change position and do the exercise five times with the right arm (left leg bent, right leg stretched).

GOOD POSTURE

Flexibility plays an important part in good posture. People with good posture signal alertness and youthfulness—no matter their biological age.

Slumping and a drooping head are two signs of old age. Both can happen for many different reasons, though biology and bad habits are the major culprits. Especially in women, the bone structure changes with age and can, in some women, result in osteoporosis, the disease that causes a person to stand and walk bent over.

Until we are about forty years old, bone mass is still generated in the body, but after this age there will be a loss in osseous tissue. In women, this happens in connection with menopause. Women aged forty-five or older lose about one percent of osseous tissue per year. Exercise with lots of movement can help reduce the loss of osseous tissue in the body. Though highly controversial, hormone replacement therapy is used by some doctors to prevent loss of osseous tissue and osteoporosis. However, hormone replacement therapy can increase the risk of breast cancer.

If bad posture is about bad habits when working or relaxing, there is only one way of improving the posture: change the habits and be conscious of standing, sitting, and walking as erectly as possible. The Dynamic Movement Exercise Program will also help improve posture.

In some cases, a "shoulder strap" can be used to stand more erect. A shoulder strap will press the shoulders back to their natural position. If bad posture is a serious problem, a specialist should be consulted.

FIRMER BREASTS

Young breasts are normally thought of as firm breasts. As with other parts of the body, the breasts also change with age—often they start to sag. How much depends upon biological age, breast size, and how much physical activity is done *without* the support of a sports bra.

Some types of sports will accelerate sagging breasts. This may be due to *not* wearing a sports bra during aerobic exercise, such as running, basketball, or similar activities where there is continuous bouncing around of the breasts. This kind of movement can end up loosening the tissue of the breasts and make them sag. Therefore, when doing any kind of aerobic exercise, a sports bra is recommended.

Some kinds of traveling, commuting, and working may put the same demands on the breasts as a workout. Through regular biking and fast walking, breasts move up and down. And as more people are on the go, this is worth paying attention to. So bras can have a preventive function. Today there are many comfortable bras that have been streamlined for a smooth look under body-hugging clothes, and new fabrics help keep the bra dry against the skin.

Short of plastic surgery, there is little to be done about breasts sagging when naked. But when clothed, a bra can help breasts look firmer. There are many different kinds of bras, for different occasions and different types of clothing. If you want a bra that will make breasts sag less, you should use the Bra Selection Guidelines.

Bra Selection Guidelines

Bra Type	What They Do	Who Should Use Them
Unlined bras Regular support, wireless	Give support to breasts	Women with non-sagging breast to prevent getting sagging breasts
Lightly lined bras Extra support, often a wire	Raise breasts	Women with moderately sagging breasts
Padded bras Extra padded bra cups, with or without wire	Give fuller breasts	Women with sagging and shrinking breasts
Push-up bras Extra support and extra padded bra cups	Raise breasts and give cleavage	Women with sagging breasts who want full-looking breasts
Separate silicone shaping bra cups	Give natural look and feel of cleavage	Women who want a discreet solution to full breasts

SMOOTHER SKIN

Just like the skin of the face, the skin of the body changes as we age. The skin on the body gets looser and more wrinkled. The wrinkling of the body is also heavily influenced by how much tanning the body has been subjected to—the more tanning and sunbathing, the more wrinkles. But also weight loss and weight gain will change the skin of the body and make it looser.

In Chapter Seven, we will look at the face, including how the sun affects the skin. The information on how to avoid the sun wrinkling the face will also apply to the body.

Unfortunately, loose skin and wrinkles are not the only biological phenomena that affect the skin of the body. Women have more fat cells on the stomach, hips, and thighs than men do, and this is the reason why many women get cellulite. Cellulite is something that is a very age revealing–phenomenon to many women.

Cellulite is fat deposits in the skin's connective tissues, which makes the skin look granulated, waffly, and bumpy. People often compare it to the skin of an orange. It is more prone to happen to women who are overweight, but because cellulite is due to hormonal changes and genetics, it can happen to all body types.

Eight out of ten women will get cellulite, which becomes more pronounced with age if not treated. And the longer the cellulite is untreated, the longer it will take to get rid of.

Getting rid of cellulite is like getting rid of other body fat—exercise and healthy eating habits are important. However, there is also a third way, massage, which affects the blood circulation. Fat tissues have the worst blood circulation, which is why fluids and waste will collect in the tissue. With a daily anti-cellulite massage in the area with cellulite, it is possible to reduce the cellulite. The massage will increase the blood circulation in the cellulite area.

While there are several options to prevent and reverse signs of aging of the body, this can be a daunting task. Luckily, there are other ways of making you, your body, and your face look younger that are just as effective. The rest of the book will focus on these options.

Anti-cellulite Massage Instruction

1. Place the leg you want to massage on a chair—make sure that you stand comfortably.

2. Start by placing both hands above the knee with the thumbs on the upper side of the thigh.

3. Press lightly and move your hands upwards, making circles or strokes.

4. When you have reached as high on the thigh as you can get, start again from the knees and move up.

5. All massaging movements must be upwards.

6. Repeat ten to fifteen times.

7. Then do the back of the thigh, and the other leg, if necessary.

8. You can use a massage cream to give a smoother massage.

The massage has to be done once a day when you start treating the cellulite. When the cellulite is gone, you can do the anti-cellulite massage every other day. You can use a hemp glove or a massage brush if your fingers are not strong enough to do 5 minutes of massage on each leg.

On your way to looking younger

❖ Staying slim has many benefits—looking younger is just one of them.

❖ You can use heels to make you look younger because tall equals young.

❖ Firm upper arms are important in signaling a youthful body.

❖ Beware of succumbing to bad posture.

4

Test Your Fashion Profile

CHAPTER FOCUS
- ❖ Style study
- ❖ Fashion attitudes
- ❖ Test yourself

The most important step on your way to looking younger is wearing the right clothes. Clothes are one of the body's big age revealers–but the great thing is, we can control this age revealer ourselves. By constantly adapting our style to what is trendy, we have countless opportunities to convey our desired visual age. But first you have to find out if your current style is sending the signals that you want to convey.

Whether we care or not, just by wearing clothes, we send signals to the rest of the world about our age. Clothing is not just about function–clothes have become very important in our communication with other people. This lifestyle aspect has become more important because we do not all wear the same type of clothing. There are many different styles, and each style sends different signals to the people around us. The one signal that matters to people who want to look younger is what the style reveals about their age.

In order to find out what your style reveals about your age, you have to identify your style preferences. This is done by taking the Style Preference Test. The test will reveal if your style is doing the job you want it to—to look younger—or if you need to make adjustments in order to wear clothes that make you look younger. The test is about the colors, patterns, fabrics, and types of clothing items that you prefer and that are normally part of your wardrobe or that represent your preferred style.

Style Preference Test

The test consists of ninety different style-related terms and descriptions arranged in ten sections. Choose one term/description in each section that best describes your style. Any particular choice does not mean that you have to wear the style, just that you like it. If you don't think that there is a term/description that fits your style, choose what comes close or skip the section.

1. Colors

a. ○ Beige
b. ○ Blue
c. ○ Pink
d. ○ Purple
e. ○ Bright colors
f. ○ Brown colors
g. ○ Faded colors
h. ○ Do not care
i. ○ What's in fashion

2. Patterns

a. ○ Do not like patterns
b. ○ Very discrete patterns
c. ○ Floral patterns
d. ○ Paisley
e. ○ Leopard patterns
f. ○ Native American patterns
g. ○ Tie-dye
h. ○ No preference
i. ○ What's in fashion

3. Fabrics

a. ○ Linen
b. ○ Tweed
c. ○ Knits
d. ○ Velvet
e. ○ Shiny fabrics
f. ○ Leather
g. ○ Sweatshirt fabric
h. ○ What's practical
i. ○ What's in fashion

4. Clothing Items

a. ○ Turtleneck
b. ○ Fur coat
c. ○ Cardigan
d. ○ Long scarves indoors
e. ○ Black nylon stockings
f. ○ Leather pants
g. ○ Cargo pants
h. ○ Sweat clothes
i. ○ What's in fashion

5. Decoration on Clothes

a. ○ Do not like decoration on clothes
b. ○ Monograms
c. ○ Bows
d. ○ Rhinestones
e. ○ Embroidery
f. ○ Fringes
g. ○ Frayed
h. ○ What's functional
i. ○ What's in fashion

6. Accessories

a. ○ None
b. ○ Pearls
c. ○ Straw hat
d. ○ Beret
e. ○ Gold jewelry
f. ○ Cowboy hat
g. ○ Bandana
h. ○ Baseball cap
i. ○ What's in fashion

7. Shoes

a. ○ Low-heeled pumps
b. ○ Shoes with bridles
c. ○ Pumps with heels
d. ○ Blunt-toed shoes
e. ○ Stilettos
f. ○ Cowboy boots
g. ○ Sneakers
h. ○ Comfortable shoes
i. ○ What's in fashion

8. Jewelry

a. ○ Don't wear jewelry
b. ○ Bracelet with charms
c. ○ Pearls
d. ○ Oversize jewelry
e. ○ Gold and diamonds
f. ○ Leather
g. ○ Organic materials
h. ○ Mix of different jewelry
i. ○ What's in fashion

9. Silhouette

a. ○ Pant suits
b. ○ Fitted skirts
c. ○ Wide skirts
d. ○ Long skirts
e. ○ Tight clothes
f. ○ Close-fitting clothes
g. ○ Baggy clothes
h. ○ Loose-fitting clothes
i. ○ What's in fashion

10. Style Preference

a. ○ Understated
b. ○ Classic
c. ○ Old-fashioned
d. ○ Sculptural
e. ○ Sexy
f. ○ Outdoorsy
g. ○ Hand-made look
h. ○ Casual
i. ○ What's in fashion

Count the number of times you have crossed off each letter (a to i) and place the numbers in the score box.

Score Box

Letters	Number of times crossed off
a	
b	
c	
d	
e	
f	
g	
h	
i	

In the Style Preference Test Key, you can learn what your style preference is. The key divides style into two categories: static styles and dynamic styles. The styles that are static rarely change, and the styles that are dynamic change often according to trends and fashion. Generally, dynamic styles will make us look younger. Some static styles are currently neutral to age, and some will make the wearer look older.

Often people dress in a mix of static and dynamic styles. Or some may prefer one style at one time and another style at other times. But, generally, many people prefer to dress in a style that is similar or somewhat similar to one of the nine styles presented in the Style Preference Test.

When we want to look younger by using the way we dress, we have to focus on the dynamic styles. These are the styles that hold the most youthful signals simply because they represent styles that are changing. If you want to look young, you have to change your way of dressing from time to time because whenever there is a new generation of young people, they create new styles of dress–and their styles have the strongest youthful signals.

Style Preference Test Key

If you have an equal distribution of choices, you can either go through the test again and be more critical of your answers or choose the key answer that you feel best resembles your actual style.

- Only or mostly a's: Your style preference is for sporty clothing and/or a minimalist style in clothing. This is a static style, but this style is mostly neutral to age.

- Only or mostly b's: Your style preference is classic. This style is static and is not optimal if you want to look younger. You should adjust your style to a more dynamic style that will help you look younger.

- Only or mostly c's: Your style preference is romantic. This style is static and is not optimal if you want to look younger. You should adjust your style to a more dynamic style that will help you look younger.

- Only or mostly d's: Your style preference is bohemian. This style is static and is not optimal if you want to look younger. You should adjust your style to a more dynamic style that will help you look younger.

- Only or mostly e's: Your style preference is glamorous. This is a static style but this style is mostly neutral to age, unless it is hip hop glamorous, which is youthful.

- Only or mostly f's: Your style preference is what can best be described as rugged or outdoorsy. This is a static style, but this style is mostly neutral to age.

- Only or mostly g's: Your style preference is what can best be described as organic and/or street style. This is a static style, but this style is mostly neutral to age.

- Only or mostly h's: Your style preference is very casual or practical/functional. This style is static and is not optimal if you want to look younger. You should adjust your style to a more dynamic style that will help you look younger.

- Only or mostly i's: Your style preference is trendy. This means that the style is very dynamic and signals a youthful style.

Today, it makes a lot sense to dress in a style that matches the age that we feel. If you are fifty years old but feel forty, this should be reflected in the way you dress. But how does a forty-year-old woman dress? Or, for that matter, how does a woman in her twenties, her thirties, her fifties, or her sixties dress? It is obvious that even though some women are the same age, they do not necessarily dress in the same way; however, there are some typical ways of dressing for each age.

In the next chapter, you will be guided on how to find the current season's style that is right for you, based on your desired visual age.

On your way to looking younger

❖ Pay a lot of attention to your style.

❖ Use clothes to make yourself look younger.

❖ Accept that your style has to change from time to time.

5

Dress Your Desired Visual Age

CHAPTER FOCUS
- ❖ Focus on trends
- ❖ Age-specific styles

Understanding the principles and influence of trends means that we have the knowledge to dress in a way that many people consider fashionable, stylish, and youthful. By associating ourselves with current fashion trends, we can send some very youthful signals about ourselves. By following the guidelines in this chapter, you can easily get the style that matches your desired visual age.

More and more people are becoming aware of fashion trends—the changes in style and taste that we see at certain intervals. Many fashionable trends are first adapted by young people, and when this happens, they are worth paying attention to because clothing and all the other style elements that are under the influence of trends hold strong signals about our age.

If we want to look younger, we can use knowledge of trends from the books *Anatomy of a Trend* and *Style Eruptions* to change other people's perceptions of our age.

The new styles that end up affecting many people are first adopted by the trendsetters (who are the people who first start wearing something new). Many trendsetters are in their twenties and thirties, but also people in their forties, fifties, and sixties can be—and are—trendsetters. But the trendsetters who are in their forties, fifties, and sixties are often copying the trendsetters who are in their twenties and thirties. By doing so, they get to look much younger than other women in their forties, fifties, and sixties who do not follow what is fashionable.

Changes in fashion happen regularly. However, it is not always easy to figure out exactly which style signals what age. The best way to stay updated is by reading about fashion trends in the well-known fashion magazines.

In fashion, there are two phenomena that influence how we dress: fads and trends. When a new style appears, one of two things can happen: the style will be popular for one season and then disappear. Then it was just a fad. Or it can go on being popular for several years, and then it becomes a trend. There is a big difference between fads and trends, and this we can take advantage of when we want our clothing to reflect our desired visual age.

If we are talking about high fashion from the famous fashion brands in Europe and in North America, their style changes so fast that only a few people register that there was a new style. When this is the case, there is really no point in using their styles to signal your age because very few people will recognize them and know how to interpret them. So if we want to use clothes and accessories to our advantage in looking younger, we have to avoid the fads that will be out of fashion in a few months' time (at the time when these designers introduce a whole new style).

Though many fashion fads are adopted by young people—and could be used to signal youthfulness—they are not really reliable because six months later they will be out of style, and the rest of the world will not know what this or that style represents in terms of youthfulness. In that way, trends are much more reliable because many people will be aware of the trendy styles and know that this style represents what is new (which equals what is young).

Trends have a longer time span and, therefore, we can also better document them—and count on them to help us signal the age that we want to signal.

Trendy styles will be popular for a long time. They will not be popular with the same people all the time, but the popularity of the trendy style will flow from the trendsetters to the rest of the population during a period of time that can be anything from three to ten years.

Fashion changes, and any style photos in this book would be outdated within a couple of seasons. Therefore, you will not find any fashion photos in *Look Younger Without Surgery*. To get updated on what is fashionable, read two or three fashion magazines, either printed versions or the online versions. Choose the well-known fashion magazines to be sure to get news on what is trendy now. While there are many online fashion resources, you cannot be sure that they are right for you: the photos may be outdated or be more representative of a style in another part of the world than where you live. No matter where you live, you can trust the US, British, and French fashion magazines to be spot-on for global fashion trends.

On your way to looking younger

❖ Go for a style that matches your visual age.

❖ Avoid going for a look much younger than your self-perceived age.

❖ Be aware that you have to update your clothing style on a regular basis to radiate youthfulness.

6

Flaunting Your Youthful Image

CHAPTER FOCUS
- ❖ Accessories overview
- ❖ Jewelry inspiration
- ❖ Face piercings

Accessories are powerful visual signifiers. Even though accessories are only a part of what we are wearing, they play a much bigger part than their actual size. Accessories are popular and there are a lot more trendy and fashionable accessories to choose from than ever before. The accessories have to look good with what you are wearing but they also have to make you look the visual age you want to convey. With the right accessories, you can further flaunt your youthful image.

Clothes and accessories play an equally important part in signaling our age to others. Clothes are the basic tool you can use in communicating your visual age, and accessories can be used to refine this communication. With our clothes, we can give a very good indication of our age but often it is the accessories that underline peoples' perceptions of our age.

There are many different types of accessories. Basically, the types of accessories that are available to us are these:

- ❖ Hats
- ❖ Hairbands
- ❖ Sunglasses
- ❖ Glasses
- ❖ Earrings
- ❖ Scarves
- ❖ Necklaces
- ❖ Watches
- ❖ Bracelets
- ❖ Rings
- ❖ Bags
- ❖ Gloves
- ❖ Belts
- ❖ Stockings
- ❖ Shoes

All accessories are not equally important, either in our wardrobe or in being age signifiers. Sometimes it is better *not* to wear certain types of accessories because they may make you look older. Here is a short overview of what the different accessories can do for you when you want to look younger.

In fahsion magazines you can also stay updated on accessories that are fashionable. Style trends in accessories do not change as often as clothing trends. Women's clothing styles change from year to year but that is not the case with respect to accessories, except for shoes and sunglasses (they change every year). The other accessories categories change every 2-3 years. Even though accessories play an important part in the signals we send to other people, sometimes there are other considerations to take into account than what is fashionable:

Hats

Sun hats or caps are very important in protecting you against the sun. Hats are often used for certain occasions like weddings and funerals.

Hairbands

Hairbands are mostly of functional value.

Sunglasses

Sunglasses are important not only for protecting the area around the eyes from the sun's wrinkle-advancing rays but also because they are important in signaling your desired visual age.

Glasses

Some people need glasses to see; other people can use eyewear as a way of looking younger—if they wear the right type of eyewear. More on this in Chapter Eight.

Earrings/studs

Earrings and studs are very popular accessories that are powerful visual signifiers because they are close to the face. When women get shorter hair—as they do as they age (more on this in Chapter Nine)— wearing studs becomes popular. Earrings/studs can, of course, be worn with all hair lengths, but sometimes they tend to make the most sense with short hair.

Scarves

Scarves can have both a functional and decorative element. Go to www.lookyoungermagazine.com to find out about the status of scarves this season.

Necklaces

A necklace can complement a style, but like other types of jewelry, it can also help us look younger when the right style has been chosen. A necklace should often match earrings because they are worn relatively close to each other, and the necklace should also complement the clothing. Not all clothing will benefit from being complemented with a necklace—it depends on the current trend.

Watches

A watch sends powerful signals because most people are wearing them. (Some people are using their cell phone or music player as their watch, and this goes especially for young people.) More on watches in Chapter Eleven.

Bracelets

Bracelets can be popular accessories depending on current jewelry trends. More on bracelets in Chapter Eleven.

Rings

Rings are popular accessories but should follow the trends to effectively signal youthfulness. More on rings in Chapter Eleven.

Bags

Bags have become a very important accessory that can be used to convey your desired visual age. Go to the online StyleGuide to find out about the bags that are trendy this season.

Gloves

Gloves go in and out of fashion. More on gloves in Chapter Eleven.

Belts

In some cases, belts are part of what is fashionable, and then they should be used like other fashionable accessories.

Stockings

Nylon stockings are also under the influence of fashion.

Shoes

Shoes are perhaps the most important accessory we have at our disposal if we want to look younger. As we grow older, there is a tendency towards wearing more comfortable shoes. If comfortable shoes convey youthfulness, then this is perfect, but that is rarely the case.

FACE PIERCINGS

Face jewelry includes eyebrow piercings and nose piercings. Piercings became popular in the 1990s, and because face piercings were first adopted by young people (including many teenagers), they do hold strong signals about youth. Actually, face piercings are such strong signals for teenagers that they will not work well for someone over the biological age of forty. Face piercings are the exception to the rule that you should try to wear what young people are wearing if you want to look younger than your biological age. Also, face piercings may draw attention to wrinkles in the face that you don't want attention drawn to (if you want to convey another age than your biological age).

Rings in the belly button are also popular but because they are mostly hidden behind clothes they have no particular influence on how young you look.

On your way to looking younger

❖ Pay a lot of attention to accessories (because people observing you do).

❖ Be aware that all or most of the accessories must come from the same age group to look convincing.

❖ Avoid face piercings, as they can draw attention to parts of the face where you do not want attention.

CHAPTER

7

Facing Your Face

CHAPTER FOCUS

❖ Skin
❖ Teeth

From a distance, the body is the big revealer of age, but close up, the face becomes the major age revealer. There are several things that can be done to convey a youthful face. No matter your age, the most important thing you can do is to stop the biological age revealers from progressing. Second, there are more and more options that can help reduce wrinkles. Because teeth age much like the skin unless well taken care of, there is also guidance on how to get the most youthful smile.

With age, the skin on the face becomes thinner, drier, and more fragile. This affects the texture of the skin. One of the first signs of this change is also the most revealing sign of aging–wrinkles. Even though not all wrinkles are due to signs of aging–unless we consider smiling a lot a sign of aging–a youthful appearance of the face becomes the number one priority for many people who want to look younger.

It can be shocking to look in a mirror and see the reflection of our biological age and not our self-perceived age. Sometimes we ourselves are bothered the most by this difference–and that is a very good reason to do something about it.

To some people, cosmetic surgery is the solution to bring balance between biological age and self-perceived age. While plastic surgery can bring some remarkable changes to the face, maybe even making it more or less wrinkle-free, it is also important to be aware that wrinkle-free is not necessarily the same as young or youthful. If a person continues to use clothing and make-up that is typical of her biological age, she will not look a lot younger, just wrinkle-free.

As more and more people also know the telltale signs of women who have had facelifts, we can end up in a situation in which the facelift becomes, in a way, an age revealer in itself. People will think to themselves: "I can see she has had a facelift, so probably she is actually twenty years older than she looks." Therefore, a facelift gives the best results when used along with youthful visual age signifiers. Of course, these age signifiers are also very powerful *without* plastic surgery.

Telltale Signs of a Facelift

❖ An unusually high forehead for a woman
❖ Eyebrows unusually high on the forehead
❖ Stretched skin between eyelids and eyebrows

Wrinkles

What most people notice about aging skin are the wrinkles. There are two different kinds of wrinkles:

❖ Dynamic wrinkles: wrinkles that appear in the face when talking, smiling, grimacing, etc.
❖ Static wrinkles: wrinkles that are visible even when not moving the face

Dynamic wrinkles are wrinkles that people of almost any age have. When we smile, we get wrinkles around the eyes, or we may make a grimace that will make a wrinkle in the forehead appear.

Because faces, skin structures, skin colors, and our lives are all different, the types of wrinkles that are dynamic and those that are static will vary from face to face. Many of the wrinkles around the eyes start out being dynamic. As age progresses, there will be more and more dynamic wrinkles, and the wrinkles that used to be dynamic will become static. There are several reasons for this. One reason it that with 22 muscles around the eye and 10,000 blinks per day, this part of the skin is in constant movement. Another reason is that the outer layer of skin around the eyes is extremely thin. It measures just one fourth of the thickness of the skin on the rest of the face. The consequence is that it dries out twice as quickly as the rest of the face.

The type of wrinkles that bother people varies from person to person. But if we take a general view, there are two sub-categories of wrinkles:

❖ **Primary Age-Revealing Wrinkles**
   "Crow's feet"
   Drooping eyebrows
   Drooping eyelids
   Pouchy eyes
   Mouth wrinkles

❖ **Secondary Age-Revealing Wrinkles**
   Forehead lines
   "Worry lines"
   Nose-to-mouth wrinkles

Typical Face Wrinkles

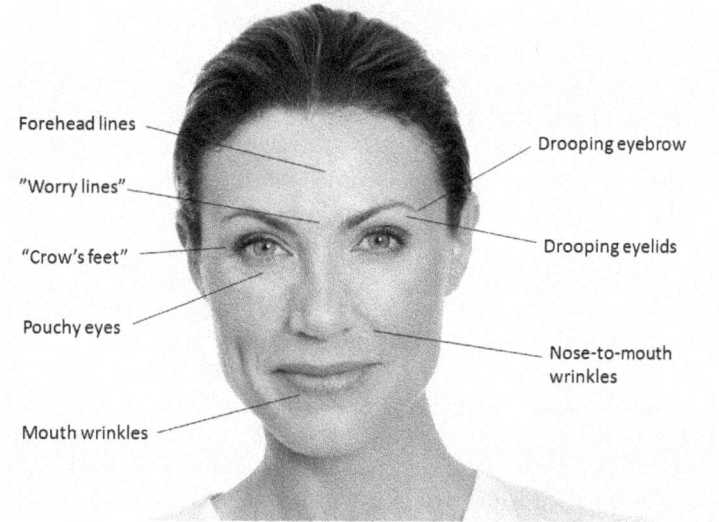

Forehead lines

"Worry lines"

"Crow's feet"

Pouchy eyes

Mouth wrinkles

Drooping eyebrow

Drooping eyelids

Nose-to-mouth wrinkles

It is often the wrinkles around the eyes that bother people the most because this area often represents the first visual change in the skin.

Today we know a lot about how and why the skin ages. A part is due to biological processes that we can do very little to reverse. But how we live our lives also affects our skin, and this we can do something about.

The skin's firmness relies on two very important connective tissue fibers, collagen and elastin. These fibers are interwoven and very elastic. They make it possible for the skin to snap back again—in the same way an elastic band will snap back—when stretched. If we want to avoid losing these tissue fibers, we have to look at what destroys the skin's collagen and elastin. Some of the collagen and elastin is destroyed in natural biological processes. But a major part of the collagen and elastin is destroyed by

❖ Sunlight
❖ Tobacco smoke
❖ Pollution
❖ Stress

Sunlight is responsible for most of the skin's aging. Dermatologists believe that the UV rays present in ordinary daylight are responsible for more than 2/3 of the skin's aging.

You can compare the aging of the skin to leaving an elastic band outside in the sun for too long. After a while, it will lose its elasticity. Exactly the same thing happens with our skin when exposed to the sun. The more exposure to the sun, the quicker the loss of elasticity in the skin.

HOW TO AVOID GETTING WRINKLES

If you want to reduce the number of lifestyle-induced wrinkles, you should do the following:

Moisturize with Sunscreen

The sun does a lot of good to sustain life on earth. So humans, animals, crops, etc., need the sun. The sun also provides vitamin D to humans, one of the vital vitamins that we do not always get enough of through food. Therefore, we cannot and should not avoid the sun altogether. However, there is no doubt that the sun causes wrinkles. Therefore, we should get as little direct sunlight as possible on the face. This is ensured by using a moisturizer containing sunscreen.

Sunscreens have different Sun Protection Factors (SPF). SPF is a numerical sunscreen rating system that is used all over the world. SPF numbers on products in stores go from 4 to more than 100. More on which SPF to use later in this chapter.

No Sun Tanning

Being tanned is not particularly youthful since people of all ages like to tan. And tanning will cause wrinkles. When you tan, this is also a sign that the sun has affected your skin in a way that also causes wrinkles. Therefore, if you want to avoid wrinkles, the basic thing is not to tan. This does not mean that you cannot stay out in the sun.

You just have to protect your skin from the sun with sunglasses, a hat with a brim, and sunscreen with the highest possible SPF. The best sunblock is non-transparent clothing. The next best is a sunscreen cream, gel, or oil. Most sunscreens should be applied 20 minutes before you go outside so that it has time to work. If you sweat a lot, the sunscreen has to be reapplied often—how often will depend on the type of product (cream, gel, or oil) and the SPF number. The lower the number, the more often the sunscreen has to be reapplied.

Avoid Direct Sunlight

The sun is damaging to the skin no matter where you are. Of course, when the sun is shining, it is not always easy to avoid direct sunlight. But staying directly out in the sun should be avoided as much as possible. If you stay out in the sun, you should, as mentioned, wear sunglasses and a sun hat or cap with a brim, and use a sunscreen with Sun Protection Factor.

The face is the part of the body that is exposed to the sun the most. However, the sun affects the skin on the body in the same way as the skin on the face. But as most people have their body covered with clothing during much of their lives, there are typically fewer sun-induced wrinkles on the body. People who sunbathe a lot or work outside unclothed without sunscreen can also get wrinkled skin on the body. Sunscreens should be used on all parts that are exposed to the sun.

When choosing a sunscreen, it is important to make sure that it filters both types of ultra-violet rays. There are two types of rays that reach the earth: UV-A and UV-B.

❖ UV-A rays penetrate deep into the skin and will destroy the skin's collagen and elastin and cause wrinkles.

❖ UV-B rays are stronger than UV-A rays; they cause redness in the skin and cause skin cancer.

Both types of UV-rays will cause you to tan, but UV-B will make the skin go red. Therefore, many sunscreens only protect against UV-B in order to avoid your skin getting red while allowing UV-A rays to pass so that the skin can tan. Sunscreen that only protects against UV-B will make your skin wrinkle.

Sunscreens with para aminobenzoic acid or cinnamates protect against UV-B rays. A sun cream, gel, or oil must contain zinc oxide, titanium dioxide, avobenzone, or benzoefurans in order to protect against UV-A rays. Also benzylidene camphor to some degree protects against UV-A rays.

If you are concerned about wrinkles and skin cancer, a sunscreen cream, gel, or oil should protect from both types of UV-rays. The information label should clearly state what kind of protection the sunscreen offers, either by stating that it contains a UV-A filter, a UV-B filter, or both. If it does not, you should find a sunscreen that clearly states what types of rays are filtered.

Darker skin types do not get sunburned as easily as lighter skin types do, but the UV-A light ages the skin in just the same way. Therefore, everybody—regardless of their skin color—should use sunscreen if they want to reduce the risk of wrinkles. In the Skin Type/Sunscreen Guidelines on the next page, you can see which SPF you should use if you do not want to get wrinkles from the sun. The guidelines clearly show that no matter what skin type you have, you should use SPF with double-digit numbers. Sunscreen rubbed on the skin will typically work for at least a couple of hours and must be reapplied according to the label instructions.

Skin Type/Sunscreen Guidelines

If preventing wrinkles is your priority, you should use a sunscreen with both a UV-A filter and UV-B filter.

Skin Type	Description	Recommended SPF
1	Very light skin, reddish hair	Minimum 80
2	Light skin, blond hair	Minimum 80
3	Olive-colored skin, brown hair	Minimum 50
4	Brown skin, dark brown hair	Minimum 50
5	Dark brown skin, black hair	Minimum 30
6	Black skin, black hair	Minimum 30

Tanning Beds

Tanning beds or similar artificial tanning devices work in the same way as the sun, and they cause wrinkles just as the sun does. How many wrinkles depends upon the tubes in the tanning bed. The tubes can transmit both UV-A and UV-B rays, or just UV-A rays or just UV-B rays. The rays have different effects on the body, as mentioned earlier. UV-A rays are the cause of wrinkles and UV-B rays are the cause of skin cancer. The kind of rays transmitted in the tanning bed is up to the owner of the device who puts the tubes in. The lettering on the tubes should reveal what kind of rays they transmit. If there is no clear indication what type of rays a tube transmits, the device should not be used under any circumstances. If you do not want to get wrinkles, you should not use tanning beds or other tanning devices.

Smoking

Tobacco smoke causes wrinkles. The tobacco contains substances that destroy the collagen and elastin of the skin.

Cigarette smoke speeds up the aging of the skin, especially at the corners of the eyes and around the mouth. Heavy smokers typically are five times more wrinkled than non-smokers who do not breathe in smoke.

If you want to reduce the number of lifestyle-induced wrinkles, you should not smoke. If you smoke, you should stop smoking. It is never too late to benefit from stopping smoking. There are several types of stop smoking aids available at drug stores if you want to stop smoking.

We know more and more about passive smoking and the perils that passive smoking contains. Passive smoking can cause cancer, cardiovascular diseases, and many other ills—as well as wrinkles. Depending upon how long you are in a smoke-filled environment and how much smoke there is, the smoke will get inside your body and do damage. If you want to reduce the number of lifestyle-induced wrinkles, you should avoid all passive smoking.

Pollution

Pollution—from exhaust fumes to factory smoke—can alter the skin because it changes how the cells in the skin divide and renew themselves. Pollution can, in fact, accelerate the production of cells that cause the ageing of the skin through a series of chemical reactions, which can end up causing wrinkles. Daily cleansing of the face with a mild soap before bedtime and using a moisturizing gel or cream in the morning are the basics of skin protection, whether you live in a polluted area or not. More than one facial or body wash with soap in 24 hours will remove the grease that the skin creates naturally as a protective barrier against pollution. If—for general hygienic reasons only—you feel the need to wash your face and/or body more than once a day, use cold water only and for as short a time as possible, and moisturize often.

Stress

Being busy and having an active life does not influence the emergence of wrinkles in any extraordinary way. But serious stress can affect the skin and also end up causing wrinkles. Stress is a physical and emotional state that is highly negative to a person's health. It can lead to depression and anxiety, which may also end up causing wrinkles. Thus, there are many good reasons to deal with stress as early as possible.

Grimacing

Smiling, chewing, and squinting can also cause wrinkles. When we use our face to express ourselves—such as smiling and grimacing—we use the elasticity of the skin. Some wrinkles are unavoidable when using our face. Smiling is important and is, in many peoples' opinion, much more appealing than an un-smiling face. But some people have habits of wrinkling their forehead or the area between their eyes and other face muscles. The more they use these face muscles, the bigger the risk of the wrinkles there becoming permanent.

If you make faces a lot and you want to avoid the wrinkles this can cause, you have to train yourself to express yourself in other ways. But first you have to become aware of what extent you make faces. You can study yourself whenever you have the chance, look at photographs of yourself, and ask people that know you if they have noticed that you make faces more than the average person.

WHAT TO DO
ABOUT WRINKLES

If you have wrinkles, there are several ways of making them less visible. What you want to do will depend upon how many wrinkles you have and where you have them. If you have age-related face wrinkles, you have the following options:

❖ Moisturizing
❖ Anti-wrinkle creams
❖ Botox
❖ Fillers
❖ Peels and scrapings
❖ Cosmetic surgery

These options work in different ways and can be used for different kinds of wrinkles. The methods can be combined. You can use the Age-Specific Anti-Wrinkle Treatment Guide to find out which biological age is *generally* relevant to the different treatments.

Age-Specific Anti-Wrinkle Treatment Guide

Biological Age Treatment	20s	30s	40s	50s	60s	70s
Moisturizing	X	X	X	X	X	X
Anti-wrinkle creams		X	X	X	X	X
Botox			X	X	X	X
Fillers			X	X	X	X
Peels and scrapings				X	X	X
Cosmetic surgery				X	X	X

Moisturizing

How we treat our skin on the outside has very little to do with getting wrinkles. Deep wrinkles are caused by the sun, tobacco, pollution, stress, and by our genes. All this causes the skin to lose its elasticity. But when we moisturize the skin, we can temporarily erase or prevent the small and very delicate wrinkles caused by dry skin from being visible. Any cream can do this, but as soon as the cream wears off or is washed off, the wrinkles will again be visible. A moisturizer is effective for less than 24 hours.

If you have small and delicate wrinkles in the face, use a moisturizer that you like, without perfume. Gels have become popular moisturizers because they do not leave the skin shiny. You should use a moisturizer that contains a sunscreen if you are often outside.

Anti-Wrinkle Creams

Most anti-wrinkle creams work in the same way as moisturizers. They will only temporarily erase the small and delicate facial wrinkles from being visible.

Anti-wrinkle creams cannot erase wrinkles permanently simply because the molecules that are supposed to erase the wrinkles cannot penetrate the skin deeply enough to affect the skin. So even if the cream contains ingredients that should work on the wrinkles, the molecules in these ingredients cannot penetrate the skin, and, consequently, cannot erase any wrinkles. The skin has a phenomenal ability to prevent outside particles from penetrating it, therefore there is no cream that can *permanently* alter the structure of the skin and erase wrinkles. Anti-wrinkle creams only affect the small and delicate wrinkles, just like a moisturizer; in fact, most anti-wrinkle creams *are* just moisturizers.

Skin-Repair Treatments Overview

Type	Description	What it Does	How it Works	Results	Side Effects
Vitamin-A acid	Cream or gel with vitamin A, which was originally used as a very effective anti-acne treatment.	Smoothes fine facial wrinkles and blotches from sun damage. It will not affect dynamic wrinkles.	Changes the cellular metabolism of the skin's surface.	Only as long as it is used.	Red, itchy, and scaling skin. Sunscreen protection essential.
Glycolic acids ("fruity acids")	Cream or facial wash with natural fruit substances.	Smoothes rough, sun-damaged skin and fades age spots.	Sloughs away dried, sun-damaged skin on the surface.	Only as long as it is used.	Red and itchy skin. Sunscreen protection essential.

There are different over-the-counter products that contain Vitamin-A acid and glycolic acids, and they are marketed under different brand names.

Botox

Botox is one of several brand names for injections that contain botulinum toxin, a poisonous substance that, when injected in certain parts of the face, can smooth wrinkles. Generally both static and dynamic wrinkles can be treated with botulinum toxin; for instance, the worry wrinkles in the forehead, between the eyebrows, and around the eyes can temporarily be smoothed by botulinum toxin.

The doses for cosmetic use are very small and are not considered dangerous. However, this does not mean that there are no risks involved. Botulinum toxin will paralyze part of the face and, if injected wrongly, it can paralyze a wrong part of the face and can cause, for instance, a drooping eyelid.

Botulinum toxin injections only take a few minutes. Normally, it takes a couple of weeks to see the full effect of the injection. Depending upon how much botulinum toxin is used, the face will lose some of its natural flexibility. The effect will last three to six months and then the treatment can be repeated.

Fillers

Fillers are injectable collagen, hyaluronic acid, or fat that can fill deep, static wrinkles, typically between the eyes, from the nose to the mouth, and on the upper lip. The filler is injected into the wrinkle where it will fill out the wrinkle.

Fillers Overview

Type	Description	Results
Injectable collagen	Collagen derived from animal or human sources	Visible right away; lasts 2-6 months
Fat	Fat from patient's own body	Visible right away; lasts up to 6 months
Hyaluronic acid	Natural component in all living organisms	Visible right away; lasts up to 1 year

The fillers are sold under different brand names. There are other types of fillers than the ones mentioned in the Fillers Overview, but they are not as well established.

All fillers may have side effects, but they are generally rare and mostly mild. When the filler has been absorbed by the body, it has to be injected again to maintain the effect.

Peels and scrapings

Peels and scrapings remove "old" skin and let new skin grow. In both peels and scrapings, the outermost layer of the skin is affected, but by different means. You can get details of the differences in the Peels and Scrapings Comparison Overview.

Peels and Scrapings Comparison Overview

Type	Description	What it Does	Results
Chemical Peel	Surgical removal of the top layer of skin with a chemical solution. Different solutions are available.	Smoothes fine and/or coarse wrinkles, depending on chemical solution used.	Visible after skin has healed.
Dermabrasion (scraping)	Scraping away the outermost layer of skin with scraping device.	Smoothes fine wrinkles.	Visible after skin has healed.
Micro-dermabrasion (scraping)	Abrasion with a fine sandblaster on outermost layer of skin.	Smoothes fine wrinkles.	Visible after skin has healed.

Treatment is performed by a dermatologist or cosmetic surgeon and normally only takes a short time. But the healing process is slow. New skin has to grow and, at first, it will be pinkish. This can be covered with make-up until the skin gets a less pinkish skin tone. This process takes several months.

At-home peeling and scrapings kits are also available, but they have no effect on wrinkles. They will clean the skin and remove the dead skin cells, something that can also be done by a sponge rub. Excessive use can have side effects, including skin diseases such as rosacea and acne.

Cosmetic Surgery

Most cosmetic plastic surgery is not about getting a more youthful look—it's about adapting to society's and/or one's own beauty ideals. This could be changing the shape of the nose or the size of the breasts. But the size of breasts or nose has nothing to do with looking younger. The size of breasts is no clear indication of age. Young people have small breasts and big breasts. Older people have big breasts and small breasts. And the same goes for noses.

But cosmetic surgery also offers options in dealing with the signs of aging, in particular in the face. And these options can be a highly effective way of getting to look more youthful. The relevant procedures are presented in the Age-Reducing Facial Cosmetic Surgery Options Overview.

Age-Reducing Facial Cosmetic Surgery Options Overview

Surgical Procedure	Target Area	What It Can Do	What It Won't Do
Forehead Lift/ Brow Lift	Forehead	Smoothes out wrinkles in forehead; lifts eyebrows and eyelids; smoothes out furrows between eyebrows.	In some cases, upper eyelids may still be drooping after surgery.
Eyelid Surgery	Upper and lower eyelids	Removes excess skin or fat on upper eyelids and/or below the eyes ("bags").	It will not remove crow's feet or other wrinkles around the eyes, eliminate dark circles under the eyes, or correct sagging eyebrows.
Facelift	Cheeks, jowls, chin, and neck	Stretches the skin in the lower part of the face; removes sagging skin and smoothes out deep creases from between the nose and mouth; removes folds and fats around the skin and neck.	It will not remove excess skin or fat around the eyes.

You can go to the Age-Reducing Facial Cosmetic Surgery Options Pros and Cons to learn a few more details about the surgical procedures and some alternatives.

A person can have a wrinkle-free face through cosmetic surgery, but surgery cannot give a youthful style and attitude. A person may have fewer wrinkles, but if the person in question has not changed the other visual signals, people will not necessarily see a younger person. In other words, cosmetic surgery is no guarantee that other people will automatically guess that a person is any younger.

Age-Reducing Facial Cosmetic Surgery Options Pros and Cons for Women

Surgical Procedure	Pros	Cons	Alternative(s)
Forehead Lift Eyebrow Lift	Can smooth out horizontal forehead wrinkles that cannot be smoothed out in any other way. Can affect two important areas at one time: horizontal wrinkles in forehead and drooping eyelids.	Risk of unhappiness with forehead area Risk of visible scars with short or thin hair Risk of infection.	Make-up, see Chapter Ten. Eyewear, learn more in Chapter Eight. Botox, learn more in this chapter Chemical peel, learn more in this chapter
Eyelid Lift	Can make eye area more youthful. There are not really any alternatives for drooping eyelids and heavy bags under the eyes.	Risk of unhappiness with eye area. Risk of visible scars with short or thin hair Risk of infection.	Make-up, see Chapter Ten Eyewear, learn more in Chapter Eight
Facelift		Does not affect small and fine wrinkles around the eyes. Risk of unhappiness with eye area. Risk of visible scars with short or thin hair Risk of infection.	Botox, learn more in this chapter Fillers, learn more in this chapter Dermabrasion, learn more in this chapter Chemical peel, learn more in this chapter

Make-up

Make-up can be used to conceal wrinkles, and trendy make-up can be used as a youthful signifier. Learn more about this in Chapter Ten.

SKIN DISCOLORATION

The color of the skin may also change as we age. Some of the color change may be "wear and tear," but there are also some changes in color that have other causes. In some cases, there are treatments available that will change the discoloration that sometimes comes with age.

Dark Circles

Dark circles under the eyes are often caused by very thin skin in the area under the eyes. The skin around the eyes is the thinnest on the face, and if a person has many visible blood vessels in this area, they can appear as purple circles under the eyes. In fact, it is blood that makes the skin dark. There are no treatments for thin skin and "dark circles" under the eyes. Make-up is the best way to disguise dark circles. More on make-up can be found in Chapter Ten.

Bags under the eyes are often due to fat deposits and/or water. As the skin loses its elasticity, the bags can get "baggy." Plastic surgery is the only way to permanently get rid of bags under the eyes. In some cases, they can be hidden by using eyewear (more on this in the next chapter).

Red Spots

Rosacea is a skin disease that causes red spots in the skin, especially on the nose, the area around the nose, cheeks, and the chin. Without treatment, rosacea may get worse over time. Other skin diseases can also become more pronounced with age or start in adult life. An unusual amount of redness in the skin, especially on the nose, should be looked at by a dermatologist. In some cases, there are treatments available that will make the redness go away.

Pigment Changes

Pigment changes can happen because of sun damage to the skin or because of hormonal changes. Best known are hyper pigmentation or brown spots. Age or liver spots are a common form of hyper pigmentation that, for many people, are signs of aging. They are the result of damage by the sun. Hyper pigmentation can occur on the face, on the neck, on the hands, and all over the body.

Hyper pigmentation can be reduced by prescription creams that lighten the skin; most contain hydroquinone, which bleaches darkened skin patches so the dark spots gradually fade to match normal skin coloration. Prescription bleaches contain twice the amount of hydroquinone, the active ingredient, as over-the-counter skin bleaches. In severe cases, there are other creams with tretinoin and a cortisone cream that a doctor can prescribe.

Hyper pigmentation can, in many cases, also be removed by laser by a medical doctor. This will not scar the skin, but a test spot in an inconspicuous place will need to be done, as laser removal sometimes make spots worse instead of better.

Broken Blood Vessels

If a person is spending a lot of time outdoors, wind, sun, and other weather influences can cause broken blood vessels in the face, in particular on the nose and on the chin.

Today, broken blood vessels can be treated with a laser. When the destroyed blood vessels are treated with a laser, they go away. After one treatment, there will be a reduction in broken blood vessels. Depending on the number and type of broken blood vessels, more than one treatment may be needed.

COLOR OF TEETH

Most people equate white teeth with youth. This is only natural because with age, our teeth often do change color. They become more yellow or grayish. There are several reasons for this. Some families have yellower teeth than the average population, and this will progress with age. In most cases, however, it is due to wear and tear. What we eat and drink and how we take care of our teeth cause the teeth to change color.

How to Avoid Getting Yellow/Gray Teeth

If you want wear and tear to affect your teeth as little as possible, there are several things you can do:

No coffee, tea, cola beverages, or red wine
All drinks, hot or cold, that contain strong color will discolor teeth if consumed repeatedly. This is true for coffee, tea, soft drinks like brown-colored cola, and red wine. Milk or water, either bottled or tap, are the best alternatives to soft drinks.

No smoking
Smoking will also discolor teeth. The more a person smokes, the stronger the discoloration. Just look into a cigarette filter to see what kind of color tobacco from one cigarette can create. Cigarette smoke will often make teeth gray.

Brushing
Brushing your teeth once every 24 hours is considered the gold standard of dental care. It must be done before going to sleep after having used dental floss. Some people do not feel fresh before having brushed their teeth in the morning after breakfast. But this cannot substitute brushing your teeth before going to sleep. Then you just have to brush your teeth twice a day.

HOW TO GET WHITER TEETH

Brushing is, of course, the everyday procedure to keep teeth and gums healthy. For general dental care, the toothpaste should contain fluoride. There is no indication that "whitening tooth pastes" will make your teeth whiter. But there are several ways a dentist can help make your teeth whiter. These are the most popular ways:

Dental Cleaning

Regular dental appointments are good for many reasons. During regular dentist appointments, the dentist can clean the outside of the teeth with extra rough toothpaste and remove tartar that can cause discoloring. Done regularly, this will help keep teeth white, though this will not make teeth bright white.

Bleaching

There are different kinds of bleaching methods. The dentist can do the bleaching at the clinic, or the patient can get a do-it-yourself kit to use at home. When done at the clinic, the patient gets a whitening gel rubbed on the teeth (set for about one hour). During that time, the dentist will use a special lamp to put light on the teeth as part of the whitening process.

At-home treatment starts with the dentist making an imprint of the teeth that is turned into soft silicone "dentures" that can be filled with a whitening gel and put in the mouth, typically overnight. This is done every night for several weeks.

Veneers

Veneers made of porcelain can be used as a new facade on teeth. To some extent, veneers can be compared to getting new enamel on the front of the teeth in the color and shape that you want. Veneers are ultra thin and very strong. If placed on a tooth correctly, they will stay in place for many years.

Gums

Receding gums are also a sign of aging. Receding gums can be a result of disease, in which case there are treatments available. If a person has receding gums, it is in some cases possible to cover the teeth with gum again. The extent to which this is possible depends on the quality and health of the gums and teeth.

Tooth Fillings

One sign of aging that is often overlooked are teeth fillings and silver and/or gold teeth. Young people have had fewer dental procedures done to their teeth because it is with age that you get dental problems that result in fillings, etc. In the twentieth-century, silver fillings and silver or gold teeth were the materials used to deal with cavities and other dental disease. This has changed dramatically—today there are other alternatives that make it harder to detect fillings and artificial teeth in the mouth. Silver fillings and metal, artificial teeth can be replaced by tooth fillings made of plastic materials.

On your way to looking younger

❖ Be aware of what makes your face age and prevent this from happening or worsening.

❖ Study your face to find out what makes you look older.

❖ Take advantage of what you can control yourself.

Visionary Cues

CHAPTER FOCUS

- ❖ Contact lenses
- ❖ Laser surgery
- ❖ Eyewear

Carefully chosen eyewear can be used to make you look younger in different ways. The design of the frame can hide age-revealing facial features, but it can also send some very youthful signals—much more so than other accessories because this accessory is worn in a way that all people you meet will notice. In other words, eyewear can effectively be used to cue people you meet as to your desired visual age.

Until we are in our forties, it is only a minority of people who need to have their vision corrected. Among those who need their vision corrected, there seem to be two schools of thought: Either you appreciate the extra style opportunities that eyewear gives you or you wear contact lenses (or get surgery). There are several reasons why many people dislike eyewear. Some cannot find frames that look good on them, many associate eyewear with getting old, and for others there are practical considerations due to their job or leisure activities.

Luckily, there are alternatives if you do not want to wear eyewear to correct your vision. But if you choose to wear eyewear, it is worth knowing that when chosen carefully, eyewear can be used to make you look younger in different ways.

The circumstances for needing eyewear or other vision correction can come early in life. Then it is either about being farsighted (you cannot read and see things at a close range) or about being nearsighted (you cannot see things at a distance). In the Vision Correction Guidelines, you can get an overview of your options to correct your vision. Some people who are either farsighted or nearsighted also have some kind of misshaping of the eye's lens. This is called astigmatism, which can also be corrected.

With age, most people need reading glasses. Many people realize when they are in their mid-to-late forties that they have trouble reading. This is due to a biological and completely natural process. In young people, the lens in the eye is soft and flexible, and readily changes shape to focus. Over time, there is a gradual hardening of the tissue making up the lens. As a result, the lens's ability to focus decreases steadily. The medical term for the reduction in eyesight is called presbyopia, but it is also popular to refer to it as "old-age vision."

People in their forties sometimes believe they have become farsighted when they suddenly find that they cannot read anything in small print but can still read street signs and watch movies comfortably. The exact cause for farsightedness is not fully known, but we know that old-age vision is the result of the lens becoming less flexible. In the Vision Correction Guidelines, you can also see what your options are if you need to have your vision corrected because of presbyopia.

Vision Correction Guidelines

Correction Method	What Can Be Corrected	Pros	Cons
Contact Lenses	Farsightedness Nearsightedness Astigmatism Old-age vision	With contact lenses, no one can see that you use vision correction. You can get contact lenses that function as reading glasses.	You may not be able to wear contact lenses at all times.
Laser Surgery	Some mild cases of farsightedness Nearsightedness Astigmatism Old-age vision (in this case, specifically a technique called Mono-vision)	After surgery, you will have "normal" vision.	Surgery can go wrong, and there's a risk that you will have to wear glasses even after surgery.
Eyewear	Farsightedness Nearsightedness Astigmatism Old-age vision	You can use glasses to your advantage in looking younger, either as an age concealer (because it hides wrinkles) or as a visual signifier.	Some types of eyewear can make you look older.

CONTACT LENSES

Contact lenses are available for almost all powers of nearsightedness correction and for many in farsightedness. There are also contact lenses that can correct mild astigmatism. Also, old-age vision can be corrected by contact lenses. They work more or less in the same way as eyeglass lenses in a frame. The contact lenses have two powers in one lens, one to correct distance vision, if that's needed, and the other to correct near vision.

Having less correction in one of the contact lenses than is actually needed is called Monovision and this often means that you can avoid using reading glasses.

LASER SURGERY

Surgery has become a popular way of correcting eyesight. Surgery is fairly safe today, but as with all surgical procedures, there is always a risk. Therefore, carefully consider your options before deciding, and always consult an experienced ophthalmologist to do the procedure. There are several techniques available today. Avoid techniques that are still considered experimental (which some operations for farsightedness are).

GLASSES

Eyeglasses consist of a frame and two lenses. If you want to use glasses, you should be aware of the signals that frames and lenses give away.

Lenses

When choosing lenses, you have two options: plastic lenses or real-glass lenses. Plastic lenses weigh less than glass, are shatterproof, and are less prone to dewing. They scratch easier, though some new plastic lenses that are hardened are less prone to scratches. Plastic lenses are thicker at higher powers, whereas regular glass is generally thinner than plastic at higher powers.

People who are nearsighted will typically also end up needing reading glasses. They will then need two different pairs of glasses— one pair for distance and one pair for reading. Or they can get one pair of glasses with lenses that correct for both near vision and presbyopia. There are two options for a combined lens: bifocals and multipower. You should always go for multipower. In bifocals, there is a rectangular area in the lenses that is used for reading. In bifocals, the reading area is very visible and reveals to others that the wearer needs reading glasses. In multipower lenses, the reading area is invisible. These lenses look just like regular glasses and will not reveal that the wearer needs reading glasses.

If you are nearsighted, thick lenses will make your eyes look smaller. If you are farsighted, thick lenses will make your eyes and everything under the lenses look bigger. This will include wrinkles and make-up.

Always make sure that you get anti-reflective coating on the lenses. This will ensure that both you and the frame look good.

Frames

The perception of glasses used to be that they made people look wiser—and also older. This is not the case anymore. Eyewear design has changed dramatically in recent years, and today eyewear has become an important accessory that can be used in different positive ways if you want to look younger. In fact, eyewear can be used to make anybody look younger, whether they need corrective lenses or not.

The right eyewear has several advantages. It can disguise wrinkles and send very youthful signals. The wrong kind of eyewear will do the exact opposite on both counts.

The most important thing is to avoid reading-glass-style eyewear, so-called half-frame eyewear. This kind of eyewear will reveal to all that here is a person who actually needs reading glasses because of aging. If you only need reading glasses, get a normal full frame with the power that you need for reading. You then use full-frame eyewear as reading glasses—they will just not look like reading glasses. Some people like half-frames because they do not have to take off the glasses when using their distance vision. With full-frames, you have to take the glasses off your nose when you're not reading. But this is the best solution with respect to camouflaging old-age vision.

EYEWEAR THAT HIDES WRINKLES

A pair of glasses can hide wrinkles around the eyes, and in some cases the eyewear can also take away attention from other parts of the face. In order to do so, you have to pay attention to the following parts of the frame:

- ❖ Size of frame
- ❖ Thickness of frame
- ❖ Placing and height of stems

Both too small and too large a frame will expose wrinkles around the eyes. Frames that are too large will also expose pouchy eyes. The thinness and thickness of the frame should be taken into consideration. Too thin a frame will not hide wrinkles.

The front of the frame is often what we pay most attention to when we choose eyewear. But the stems can also be effective in hiding wrinkles around the eyes, especially "crow's feet." Too thin a stem or a stem placed at the top of the front of the frame will not hide wrinkles. A stem that has some height will hide wrinkles.

The illustrations show variations as drawings, not real frames, on frame and stem height and placement. They show some principles but do not represent eyewear trends. However, it is important to be aware that eyewear not only can be used to conceal wrinkles, but also can be used as a visual signifier to signal youthfulness.

Too large a frame (left) and correct-sized frame to hide wrinkles

**Too thin a frame (left) and a good frame
thickness to hide wrinkles**

**Stems that are too thin (left) and stems that are
correctly proportioned and placed to hide wrinkles**

Age-Concealing Eyewear Selector Guide

Wrinkle Type	Eyewear Frame	Eyewear Color
Worry wrinkle	High nose bridge	Good match with eye color
Drooping eyebrow	Dominant upper frame	Same or similar color as eyebrows
Drooping eyelid	Small frame pointing up	Highlight eye color
Bags under the eyes	Small dominant frame	Highlight eye color
Dark circles under the eyes	Small dominant frame	Dark color

You can use eyewear whether you need prescription glasses or not. If you do not need prescription glasses, you can just have regular "window glass" as lenses.

Eyewear as Visual Signifier

Eyewear has become fashionable, and there are many trendy frames available in opticians' stores. If used properly, eyewear can be a very strong visual signifier. Eyewear is very visible—it is on the face—and if it is the right trendy eyewear, it will help communicate your desired visual age.

If you want a pair of glasses that can help you look younger, the best sources are either fashion magazines or a trendy optician's store.

Face Wrinkle Concealing Options Overview

Wrinkle Type	Options	Chapter Focusing on This Option
Forehead lines	Bangs	9
Worry lines	Eyewear	8
	Make-up	10
Drooping eyebrows	Raise eyebrow	10
Drooping eyelids	Eyewear	8
	Make-up	10
Mouth wrinkles	Make-up	10
	Cosmetic procedures	7
Pouchy eyes	Eyewear	8
	Make-up	10
Dark circles under eyes	Eyewear	8
	Make-up	10
Nose-to-mouth wrinkles	Cosmetic procedures	7
Mouth wrinkles	Make-up	10
Double chin	Slimming	3

On your way to looking younger

❖ Consider carefully your options in contact lenses and/or eyewear if you need vision correction.

❖ Pay attention to eyewear that can make you look younger.

❖ Choose lenses with invisible power lines if you are both nearsighted and need reading glasses.

CHAPTER 9

Young-Looking Hair Days

CHAPTER FOCUS
❖ Hair length
❖ Hairstyle
❖ Hair color

Hair sends very strong signals about age. Hair length and haircut are generally much more important than hair color when you want your hair to influence people's perceptions of your age. People of all ages have almost all kinds of hair colors, so hair color is not a strong signal in relation to age—except with gray hair. Knowing exactly what your hair reveals to other people makes it easy to control these signals.

Hair is an important way of signaling our self-perceived age, but it also has some limitations compared to clothing and accessories. Almost any woman can dress in fashionable clothes and choose to wear trendy make-up, but changing one's hair according to trends or certain popular hairstyles is not always an option. Maybe one's hair type is not right for a certain haircut, or the hair is too short to change into a hairstyle with long hair (even though hair extensions can make up for that).

So, while it is not possible for everybody to change hair length or have the most desirable hairstyle or hair color, most people have at least one of the options, and many will have two of these options available to them.

HAIR LENGTH

Women with longer hair look younger. This perception is clearly related to the fact that more younger women than older women have long hair (anything from shoulder-length hair to elbow-length hair). Women get shorter hair as they get older for many reasons:

- ❖ Short hair is (sometimes) less time-consuming to care for.
- ❖ Short hair for women over 30 is a long tradition.
- ❖ Hair stylists push for shorter haircuts because there is more money to be made with hair that needs to be cut often.
- ❖ Women's hair gets thinner and finer with age.
- ❖ Gray hair gets more attention when long, and women who do not color their hair sometimes want to avoid that.

With age elasticity and women feeling younger longer, it is obvious that the age when women cut their hair short will also change. Women will have longer hair for a longer time, maybe even well into their fifties. And this is the right approach if you want to look younger. It is not about getting the longest hair possible, but having a hair length that signals the visual age you want to convey. You can use the Age Group/Hair Length Guidelines to find the hair length that will match your desired visual age.

Age Group/Hair Length Guidelines

Age Group	Youthful Hair Lengths That Represents Each Age Group
Look like someone in her 20s	Upper arm length or longer
Look like someone in her 30s	Upper arm length to shoulder length
Look like someone in her 40s	Shoulder length or shorter
Look like someone in her 50s	Neck length or shorter
Look like someone in her 60s	Short hair

As already mentioned, long hair may not be an option for everybody, and then the right thing to do is focus on style and color. But if you would like to have longer hair and are impatient for your hair to grow, you can use hair extensions that are connected to your own hair. A specialized hair stylist will be able to integrate hair extensions into your own hair so that no one will notice that you have hair extensions. You can get extensions in more than fifty different hair colors, which can be mixed according to your natural hair color. The best hair extensions are made with real hair, which also means that the extensions can be treated like regular hair. The hair extensions can be colored, and curling irons, curlers, and the like can be used just as with your own hair.

HAIRSTYLE

Bangs are mostly popular with young people, and, therefore, bangs do convey a youthful look in themselves. With a trendy haircut, the youthful signals can be even stronger. Bangs have the following characteristics:

- ❖ They can be used to hide wrinkles on the forehead
- ❖ If very low, they can be used to hide drooping eyebrows
- ❖ They often signal a young age
- ❖ They are not always in fashion

Basically, bangs have several things going for them if you want to look younger. This does not mean that they are the right solution for everybody. Bangs do not look good on all women, and some women have hair that will not do the trick of hiding wrinkles.

If we look back through the past few decades, we can easily see that different hairstyles were popular at different times. At each decade, there were certain hairstyles that were popular and are now considered typical of the period. Some women stick to the same hairstyle for decades, and they may end up having a hair-do that is representative of a decades old hairstyle. For a youthful look, it is important to choose hairstyles that are current no matter the age you want to convey.

Age-Specific Hairstyles

What visual age do you want to convey with your hairstyle? You may want to convey the same age as in clothing and accessories—or a slightly different age. Some women will want their hair to convey an age that is older than their visual age for clothing—and for other women, it will be the opposite. The *Look Younger Magazine* Hair Guide keeps you updates about age-specific hairstyles.

HAIR COLOR

Some people may have preferences for blonde, or brown, red, or black hair, but when it comes to hair color, specific hair colors do not convey certain ages. All hair colors can look equally young—except for gray or grayish hair. If you do not have gray or grayish hair, there is no age-related reason to dye your hair.

Hair color is not as much under the influence of trends as haircuts. Also, young women do not dye their hair nearly as often as older women. There can be many reason why a woman wants to dye her hair, but unless her hair is gray or grayish, to look younger should not be one of them.

Gray or grayish hair is one of the biggest age revealers that we know. And getting graying hair happens to most people when they are old enough. But people can get gray hair at any age after thirty.

How early we start getting gray hair is determined by our genes. This means that most people will start getting gray hairs around the same age that their parents and grandparents first got their gray hair. From the time a person notices a few gray hairs, it may take more than ten years for all of that person's hair to turn gray. Gray hair is more noticeable in people with dark hair because it stands out, but people with light hair are just as likely to get gray hair.

The cause of gray hair is well known. The root of every strand of hair is fastened in a hair follicle. Each hair follicle contains a certain number of pigment cells (as does the skin). The pigment cells continuously produce a chemical called melanin (as does the skin) that gives growing hair its color of blonde, red, brown, black, etc. The dark or light color of someone's hair depends on how much melanin each hair contains.

As we get older, the pigment cells in the hair follicles gradually die. When there are fewer pigment cells in a hair follicle, the hair will no longer contain as much melanin and will become a more transparent color—like gray, silver, or white —as it grows. As we get older, there are fewer pigment cells to produce melanin. Eventually, the hair will be completely gray.

Luckily, gray hair is also one of the easiest hair issues to do something about—with hair dye. Use the Age-Concealing Hair-Dyeing Guidelines for the best results. If you have gray or grayish dyed hair, you should consider dyeing your hair into your own original hair color or get a salt-and-pepper color.

Skin Tone and Hair Color Matching Guide

Generally, the hair color should only be one to three shades different from the skin tone. If in doubt about the natural color of your hair, you can use the Skin Tone and Hair Color Matching Guide, which (in grey tones) tell you that the darker the skin tone, the darker hair color will look natural.

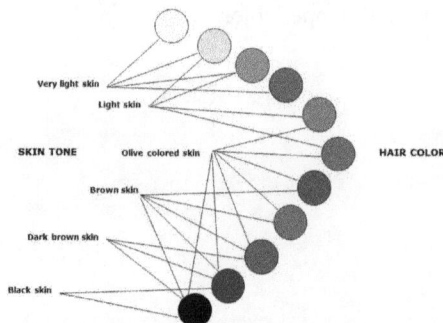

Very light skin
Light skin
SKIN TONE
Olive colored skin
Brown skin
Dark brown skin
Black skin
HAIR COLOR

Hearing Aids

For some people, a loss of hearing is part of growing old. About fifteen percent of people between the biological ages of sixty and eighty will have some kind of hearing loss. For some, the reduction of hearing will warrant a hearing aid early in life, but for most people a hearing aid is only needed late in life. If a hearing aid is warranted, you will want to conceal it, of course. Technology has changed the shape and the design of hearing aids dramatically since the beginning of the twenty-first century. Today, there are many options, and the right hearing aids for people who want to look younger are miniscule and hidden inside the ear. Otherwise, hairstyle plays an important role in hiding a hearing aid.

Hair Bands

If you have long hair, hair bands and hair slides often come in handy. Hair bands can be scarves worn as hair bands or regular hair bands of metal or plastic.

Hats

Has are worn for functional and decorative reasons. Out in the sun, however, it is important to wear a hat or cap if you want to protect yourself from the sun's rays. Of course, out in the cold it is also important to wear a hat. At special occasions, such as weddings and funerals, hats are sometimes worn. Hats can also be part of what is fashionable, and then certain styles of hats will be popular.

Wigs

Whether you wear a wig or not is not what determines your age. It's the hairstyle or the style of the wig. The same style that signifies certain ages for real hair also applies to wigs.

On your way to looking younger

❖ Long hair will make you look younger.

❖ Gray hair colored into salt and pepper or your original hair color generally looks the most convincing.

❖ Make sure that people cannot see that you color your hair.

CHAPTER **10**

Using Make-up the Youthful Way

CHAPTER FOCUS
- ❖ Concealing one's age
- ❖ Trendy make-up

Make-up is the classic tool for disguising a woman's age. But using make-up in itself is no guarantee that you'll look younger. It is about using the right style of make-up and the right colors. This is because various make-up colors and various make-up styles convey very different signals about age. If you want to use make-up that conveys youthful signals, you have to wear make-up that is trendy.

Women have many different approaches to make-up—from wearing nothing to using a lot of make-up. There may be different reasons for not wearing make-up, but used moderately, make-up can really help many women look younger.

A lot of make-up does not necessarily conceal age. Sometimes it will actually make other people aware that you wear make-up and make them conclude that this is done in order to camouflage age.

Also, make-up in itself does not necessarily make someone look younger. Some women find a certain make-up that they like and will apply the same kind of make-up year after year after year. If they do not realize that make-up styles change over time, they will end up applying a make-up style that is outdated, and people will think, "Why is she wearing make-up that makes her look older?"

But make-up can help women look younger, and there are two very different ways that this can be done:

❖ Make-up can conceal age-related facial changes.

❖ Make-up trends can be used as visual age signifiers.

This chapter has two sets of guidelines that each represent one of these options. You can choose to use only one of the guidelines or both. When studying the two guidelines, there may be options that will be contradictory. This is because what works best to conceal a certain age may not be what is trendy.

Both guidelines are inspirational guides that take into account that people have different facial features and different skin tones. Because it is impossible to give detailed instructions for all face types, the guides give only principle instructions. There is no general advice on how to apply make-up, and there are no recommendations of any particular make-up brands. You can choose a brand that you like, that works well with your skin type, and that fits your budget.

Using Make-up to Conceal Age

Concealing wrinkles with make-up

Forehead lines

Drooping eyebrow

"Worry lines"

"Crow's feet"

Drooping eyelids

Pouchy eyes

Nose-to-mouth wrinkles

Mouth wrinkles

Sometimes Possible to Conceal with Make-up

❖ Drooping eyebrows
❖ "Crow's feet"
❖ Pouchy eyes

Rarely Possible to Conceal with Make-up

❖ Forehead lines
❖ "Worry lines"
❖ Drooping eyelids
❖ Nose-to-mouth wrinkles
❖ Mouth wrinkles

The basic elements in age-concealing make-up are concealer sticks and foundations. A concealer stick is used on smaller areas that need the most coverage, while foundation is used on larger areas. Normally, the concealer stick is used first before foundation is rubbed on the skin on top of the area covered with concealer stick.

Concealers are thicker and more opaque than regular foundation makeup. A concealer will not work well on the thin, delicate skin around the eyes, since it will often collect in the creases. In this area, you should use a normal fluid foundation. And if you use the foundation during the day, it should have a high Sun Protection Factor (SPF); a waterproof concealer has obvious advantages.

The important thing to remember is that while it is easy to use a concealer stick and foundation to cover skin completely, this does not necessarily make anyone look any younger. When other people can see that a lot of concealing make-up has been used, they may automatically think that this must be someone older since she needs to use all that make-up. Concealing make-up should not cover any more skin than absolutely necessary; this will make the skin look natural—like someone who does not need cover make-up.

The key to looking as natural as possible is to pick a concealer stick and a foundation that looks exactly like your complexion without any make-up. Before you buy a concealer stick or foundation that you have not used before, you should always try it on your facial skin first.

The best way to find the concealer stick and foundation is to put three to five foundations on the skin of your face at the same time. Then you will typically see that there are differences in the color of the foundations, and you can pick the one that is most like your complexion. If the first three to five you try are not exactly right, you should try on three to five more. If you have a pale complexion and cannot find a foundation that is exactly like your skin color, go for one that is lighter rather than darker. The opposite is the case if your complexion has a little bit of color—then you should go for a foundation that is darker rather than lighter. Also remember to choose a foundation that is matte if your complexion is generally not shiny. If your complexion is shiny, you can consider a more radiant tone to the foundation.

The concealer stick should also be the same color as your complexion and the foundation. And the same guidelines in choosing a foundation apply to concealer sticks. If you can find a concealer the exact same color as your skin tone, you may not have to use a foundation on top of it.

As mentioned, neither concealer stick nor foundation should be used to cover more skin than absolutely necessary. By choosing a concealer stick and foundation in the same color as your complexion, you don't have to cover skin that does not need covering. And skin that is not covered with make-up will always look more natural than skin covered with make-up.

Age-Concealing Make-Up Guidelines

Find the wrinkle type that you want to conceal. Read the accompanying make-up suggestion. Do not use more make-up than necessary.

Wrinkle Type	Make-up Suggestions
Forehead lines	Strong focus on mouth will take attention away from forehead.
Worry lines between the eyebrows	Often eye shadow will draw attention to this area.
Drooping eyebrows	Sometimes you can "elevate" eyebrows using make-up. See boxed text on how to lift your eyebrows.
Drooping eyelids	Make upper lashes as long as possible, and make them turn up. Brush eye shadow upwards to sides. Keep it toned down.
Crow's feet	Strong focus on lashes without looking "made-up." Brown or dark gray mascara will often work best to accomplish this. Gray is best for pale skin, whereas brown is better for a "warm" complexion.
Pouchy eyes	Make both upper and lower lashes as long as possible.
Dark circles under eyes	Use concealer stick before foundation. Apply a little eye shadow in a skin tone under the eyes.
Mouth wrinkles	Use lipstick pencil to prevent lipstick from running. Lipstick and lipstick pencil must be same color.
Discoloration, etc.	Use concealer sticks and foundations that look natural to your skin tone.

Age-specific Make-up Guidelines

With make-up, you can convey the same age that you do with your clothing and accessories, or a different age. Some women will want their make-up to convey an age that is younger or older than their desired visual age in other categories. You can use the Age-specific Make-up Guidelines to find out what is right for you.

Product Age Group	Mascara* *(must look natural in relation to eyebrows and hair colors)*	Eyeliner (if in fashion)	Eyebrow Pencil	Lipstick/ Lipstick Pencil
20s	Black	Should match mascara.	Color that enhances eyebrow color.	
30s	Black	Should match mascara.	Color that enhances eyebrow color.	
40s	Black	Should match mascara.	Color that enhances eyebrow color.	Lipstick pencil will prevent lipstick color from feathering, "bleeding," or otherwise migrating into the skin around the lips.
50s	If warm skin tone, use dark brown mascara. If pale skin tone, use dark gray mascara.	Should match mascara;	Color that enhances eyebrow color.	Lipstick pencil will prevent lipstick color from feathering, "bleeding," or otherwise migrating into the skin around the lips.
60s	If warm skin tone, use dark brown mascara. If pale skin tone, use dark gray mascara.	Should match mascara;	Color that enhances eyebrow color.	Lipstick pencil will prevent lipstick color from feathering, "bleeding," or otherwise migrating into the skin around the lips.

Skin-type Adjustments Guidelines

Consult the Skin-type Adjustment Guidelines to adjust the trendy make-up colors to your specific skin type. Make sure that the trendy result makes you look and feel good.

Skin type 1: Very light skin, reddish hair	Choose lighter version of colors
Skin type 2: Light skin, blond hair	Choose lighter version of colors
Skin type 3: Olive-colored skin, brown hair	No adjustments
Skin type 4: Brown skin, dark brown hair	No adjustments
Skin type 5: Dark brown skin, black hair	Choose stronger versions of some or all colors
Skin type 6: Black skin, black hair	Choose stronger versions of some or all colors

Usually, adjustments do not have to be made for eye color, though very light-colored eyes may work best with more discreet make-up colors.

If you color your hair, you may also want to color the eyebrows. They should be colored one shade lighter or darker than the hair. This will make the make-up look more natural.

Eyebrow Lift with Make-up

In many cases, you can use an eyebrow pencil to visually lift your eyebrows. It is up to you to decide which shape you want—for instance, full at the center and thinning towards the sides. You will probably get the best result if you keep the natural shape of your eyebrow. If you normally remove hairs on the upper side of the eyebrow, you should let them grow out before visually lifting your eyebrow.

What to use

- ❖ A pair of slanted tweezers
- ❖ An eyebrow pencil in the color of your eyebrows, or one shade darker
- ❖ A close-up mirror

How to visually lift an eyebrow

- ❖ Color the upper half of the eyebrow (where there are hairs) with an eyebrow pencil so you know where *not* to remove hair.
- ❖ Start slowly—at the side—with the tweezers to remove hairs at the lower part of the eyebrow (that is, the part that has not been colored).
- ❖ It is important that the eyebrow is not too thin at the sides (so that it "disappears").
- ❖ Continue to remove hair from the lower part of the eyebrow, but do it so that you leave more and more hair towards the eyebrow closest to the nose.
- ❖ Color the rest of the eyebrow with the eyebrow pencil.
- ❖ If the eyebrow is too thin, use the eyebrow pencil to add a little color on the skin *above* the eyebrow.
- ❖ The final result should look as natural as possible.

Using Make-up to Look Younger

When looking for make-up that signals a certain age, get inspiration from the general trends in make-up, not from what is faddish for one season with maybe just one brand. Make-up that looks youthful follows major trends in make-up.

The cosmetics companies that promote different new looks each season can be compared to fashion houses promoting a certain style for just one season. As with clothing styles, only a small number of people will get to know these looks. Only make-up trends that many people understand will help signal the desired visual age. Using make-up to look younger is about following the long-term trends, not fads.

On your way to looking younger

❖ Use make-up that conceals your age.

❖ Don't use more covering make-up than absolutely necessary.

❖ Use trendy make-up colors.

Moving Signals

CHAPTER FOCUS

- ❖ Skin
- ❖ Nails
- ❖ Jewelry
- ❖ Watches
- ❖ Tattoos

Our hands and feet are not major factors when people decode our age, but they can be the final touches that can leave no one in doubt about the age we want to convey. Turning hands and feet into visual signifiers is not difficult. Therefore, hands and feet are worth taking into account, both the cosmetic options and accessories, with jewelry that adorns fingers and wrists.

Hands play a significant part in our non-verbal communication with other people. Therefore, hands get their fair share of attention when we interact with other people. Generally, people look at hands simply because they are the part of the body most commonly used to touch other people. When we are intimate with another person, the hands can play a significant role. But this does not mean that the hands are a part of the body that we generally look to for clues about someone's age. When people—and in particular women—pay attention to the hands, it is often because of the decorative possibilities: nail polish, finger rings, bracelets, and watches.

SKIN

The skin of the hands is like all other skin affected by age. There is some wear and tear because we use the hands a lot. But hands are also often exposed to the sun, which creates wrinkles unless the skin is protected with sunscreen.

A cream with sun block is the basic way to avoid wrinkles on the upper side of the hands. Wearing gloves could do the same, but today, gloves are generally not worn, except at certain occasions, such as weddings and funerals in certain circles. A sports glove can be a good investment if you do a lot of sports using the palms of your hands or do sports outdoors. A sports glove will also keep the skin from getting callused.

Young women have callus-free soles of the feet when barefoot or wearing sandals because callused skin under the feet becomes more pronounced with age. As we age, it becomes more important to remove calluses on a regular basis. Well-cared-for feet are the best way to convey youthfulness with your feet.

NAILS

For some women, well-cared-for hands and feet are also about nail polish. Some people find painted nails beautiful, and painting nails is especially worth doing when the nails change color because of age; nails typically get more yellow.

Like other kinds of cosmetics, nail polish is also affected by trends. Fashion magazines will also update you on make-up trends.

JEWELRY

Finger Rings

Most women who are married wear a wedding ring. This you should wear no matter the style or what is says about your age. The important signal here is that you are married! But for all other rings, be aware that they are fashion accessories that are under the influence of trends. Not just the style but also the number of rings is under the influence of trends.

Toe Rings

Wearing rings on your toes has been popular at different times. Go to www.lookyoungermagazine.com to find out what the current status of toe rings is.

Bracelets

Bracelets, both style and the number of bracelets, are under the influence of trends.

Ankle Bracelets

Like toe rings, ankle bracelets have been popular at different times.

Watches

Watches are practical and essential to many people, not only because they tell the time but also because they can be used to underline one's style. A watch is, of course, an accessory, and to some, a piece of jewelry. But watches are also an important conveyer of age.

Tattoos

For decades, tattoos were in the sole domain of men, in particular, sailors and bikers. In the 1990s, tattoos became more widespread among men, and also among women. In particular, many young women got a small tattoo. It might be on the back, on the shoulder, or at the ankle. Though tattoos have been popular with the young age groups, this does not mean that the rest of the world interprets tattoos as young or youthful, at least not when it comes to women. Tattoos are also trendy, and because style changes, it is often best to avoid something as permanent as a tattoo.

On your way to looking younger

❖ If you use nail polish, it should be in a trendy color.

❖ Make sure that the jewelry you wear fits with your overall look.

❖ A watch is an important accessory as a visual signifier.

CHAPTER 12

Fragrances for Any Age

CHAPTER FOCUS
- ❖ Trendy fragrances
- ❖ Age-specific fragrances

Has fragrance anything to do with how young we look? No and yes. Fragrance has something to do with how youthful we *smell*. As there are also trends in fragrance, a fragrance can be used to highlight the signals we are sending with our clothes, accessories, hair, etc. Using the fragrance guide in this chapter, you have a chance to find a fragrance that will underline—and not undermine—your desired visual age.

Movies, magazines, and television cannot tell us how the young people we watch or read about smell. But as fragrance has become so common to use, there is no doubt that fragrance plays an important part in the signals we send. And as with other items that contain an element of style and taste, there are different choices, and some fragrances will be preferred by certain age groups. If we can identify the preferred fragrances for each age group, we have one more tool at our disposal when we want to radiate youthfulness.

Fragrance Basics

Fragrances are typically categorized into these six groups:

Citrus: Scents from citrus fruits, such as lime, lemon, tangerine, and mandarin. These are refreshing and light.

Green: Grassy scents with pine, juniper, and leaves. Have a sporty aroma.

Mossy: A combination of fresh herbs and mossy ferns. Have a strong and fresh aroma.

Woodsy: A notably woodsy-mossy mix with hints of bergamot, oak moss, and patchouli. Have a sweet and earthy aroma.

Floral: Scents from flowers, such as roses, orange blossoms, gardenias, jasmine, and carnations. The smell is like standing in a floral boutique.

Oriental: A mix of spices, amber, balsams, and resins. Has a heavy, musky scent.

Trends in fragrance change just as trends in fashion do. In the 1990s, citrus became very popular and was what young people preferred. Floral scents are widely popular with women of all ages. The heavy, oriental aromas are the opposite of the citrus scent, which meant that in the 1990s, this scent was not youthful at all.

The length of time the fragrance has been on the market often plays a part in how trendy it is. Some women fall in love with certain fragrances when they are first introduced and buy them again and again, even for decades if the particular fragrance is still available. Therefore, fragrances that have been on the market for years will often be preferred by older women, whereas new fragrances may be just getting their following among young women who may become fans for life, just as older women have become fans with the older fragrances.

On your way to looking younger

❖ Fragrances can be used to send signals about age.

❖ Avoid fragrances that have been on the market for decades.

Lifestyle Accessories

CHAPTER FOCUS
- ❖ Cell phones
- ❖ Cameras
- ❖ Music players
- ❖ Laptops
- ❖ Luggage

More and more objects are not only about functionality but also about style. When style becomes part of a product category, we start interpreting the design as we do with fashion—something that sends out different signals, including the age of the person using the products. This means that you have to pay attention to the style of the products that you use. Some products are perceived as more youthful than others are. Here is an overview of product categories where style plays a role.

Most people are not aware of it, but today we have more possibilities of signifying youthfulness than ever before because of the so-called lifestyle accessories. The term "accessory" is changing; rather, what are considered accessories is changing. There are the traditional accessories, such as sunglasses, bags, and shoes. Now there are also lifestyle accessories, for instance, cell phones, music players, and suitcases. These are designed products that can also be used to send youthful signals.

There are many different types of products to choose from in the lifestyle categories. Identifying the products that are appealing to young people is partly about identifying what is new and innovative, but it's not only that. There are many reasons for certain preferences in lifestyle products, and some have to do with how young people live their lives. But anybody who wants to underline their youthfulness can use lifestyle products, as long as they choose the right ones.

Though they are not as age-specific as other accessories, there certainly are some lifestyle accessories that work better than others. Here is an overview of five different lifestyle accessories categories that are heavily influenced by style:

Cell Phones

More and more people are using cell phones, and there are many to choose from. This means that it is important to choose a model that has a stylish and innovative look.

Cameras

Most people now use their cell phones as cameras and we rarely have a camera with us except for special occasions and holidays. But when we do have a camera, it is important that it helps you underline the age that you want to convey.

Tablet computers

If you use a computer, there are many to choose from, not least of which is the portable kind. Many people also use a tablet computer. They, too, can convey some powerful, youthful signals.

Luggage

Luggage with wheels is very practical and is why people of a certain age started using suitcases and carry-ons with wheels. Now, everybody is using luggage with wheels simply because it makes traveling so much easier. But it is important to choose, for instance, trolleys that do not make you appear any older than you are.

On your way to looking younger

❖ If you use lifestyle accessories, be aware that they also signal age.

❖ Choose lifestyle accessories that are fairly new to the market.

❖ If you want to use lifestyle accessories to help underline your desired visual age, you have to change them at certain intervals.

Cues for the Young Mind

CHAPTER FOCUS
❖ Personality
❖ Life phases
❖ Music
❖ Books
❖ Movies

With all the effort you put into looking younger than your biological age, why not also nourish a youthful mind? It is worth remembering that, to some people, it is the age of the mind that truly reveals a person's age. To take advantage of this, we have to be aware that our interests and conversations change as we grow older; make sure that you can share interests and conversation not only with people your own age but also with people whose biological age matches your self-perceived age.

Our body and face change as we age, but there is one thing that does not change—our personality. Psychological research has documented that the basic traits in our personality do not change a lot over time.

Our personality is, to a great extent, fully developed by our early twenties. If, at twenty, you are extroverted and speak rapidly, you are likely to be the same at seventy. And if you are modest and insecure when you are twenty, then it is not very likely that this will have changed when you are forty.

So, while our looks change as we age, we have a stable core inside— our personality—that is not likely to change dramatically once it is fully developed. This is the conclusion drawn from a number of studies in which scientists have observed the same group of people for several decades. In several of the studies, more than thirty years passed between the first and the last personality tests.

PERSONALITY AND AGE

One study was begun in the 1930s. Back then, a group of high school students was interviewed for a long-term study of personality traits. When they were twenty years old, they were interviewed a second time. The third interview took place when they were in their mid-thirties, and the final one when they were forty-five years old. During each interview, they were asked about their attitudes towards life, and, depending on the subject's age, parents, teachers, or spouses were also interviewed about the subject's personality at that particular time in his or her life.

Clinical psychologists made personality charts for each individual and continually analyzed the results. The scientists tested ninety different character traits for each subject, and in all cases there was a close personality resemblance between individual subjects in high school and the same person three decades later. Lively and optimistic teenagers had the same positive attitude in their forties. And individuals who had been very moody in high school were just as moody as adults.

In another study, psychologists from the National Institute of Aging in Baltimore, Maryland, studied several hundred men from the time they were about twenty-five years old until they retired. Based on the subjects' responses to a number of hypotheses and questions, they were placed in different categories: insecure, anxiety-prone, co-dependent, etc. This study confirmed the hypothesis that the personality an individual exhibits in his or her early twenties will not change for the rest of his or her life.

Another study of personalities focused on middle-aged and elderly people. Back in 1947, scientists at the University of Minnesota tested seventy-one men in their fifties. Thirty years later, the same group of men was tested again. The conclusion: their personality traits had not changed. There was, for instance, no change in the degree of extroversion and introversion during the thirty-year time period. The fifty-year-olds who had been sociable and self-assured had precisely the same traits when they were eighty.

OUR PERSONALITY DOES NOT CHANGE WITH AGE

In another study from the University of California at Berkeley, the researchers were interested in studying the development in women's personalities over time. A group of psychologists interviewed fifty-three women when they were thirty years old, and again when they were seventy years old. This study confirmed the other studies: there were no changes in, for instance, extroversion, irritability, or happiness. Women who were grumblers when they were thirty were grumblers throughout their adult life.

Few psychologists will conclude that no changes take place in personality over time for all people—it is just not the norm. Illness, such as depression, can have an enormous influence on one's personality, as can stressful situations, such as unemployment, divorce, or the death of a close family member. But there is a difference between short-lived changes in behavior and personality and fundamental and definitive changes in personality.

This is good news for all who are happy about their personality (or whose family and friends are happy with it). Some things do not change, and we do not have to worry about an "aging personality."

The studies do not claim that people do not change at all psychologically. It is only natural that our needs, interests, and attitudes change with age. That change often seems to go in a certain direction—we become more conservative. Not necessarily in the political sense of the word, but in the sense that we have "figured everything out" and maybe we are not as flexible in our needs, interests, and attitudes as we used to be.

Being conservative in the non-political sense of the word can be quite counterproductive to a youthful image. The young mind is—generally speaking—more open-minded, curious, and excited by new things (of all kinds). A person who is open-minded, curious, and excited by new things, therefore, will underline youthful signals.

The consequence is not a change in your personality (which is not really an option, anyway). But people will perceive you as being younger if you are able to relate to topics and issues that people younger than you relate to or are interested in. Then people who are younger than you will be interested in talking to you and hearing your opinion. Being associated with people who are younger than you—in one way or another—will also reflect on you and make you appear younger, too.

A young mind—no matter the biological age of the mind—is curious about many things. It is not about changing one's own preferences and dislikes but being aware that there are other tastes—and being open-minded to other people's tastes.

You can learn a little bit or have your memory refreshed by listening to music, reading books, and/or seeing movies that young people are interested in or that describe what it is like to be young.

AGE-SPECIFIC MUSIC GENRES

One thing that is a big age revealer is music. The older generation generally does not like the music that young people like. This has been the situation for decades and is not likely to change. But the generations' taste in music does change. Music changes all the time—a fact that can spark many discussions between the generations about musical taste.

There is no doubt that some people who listened to a certain kind of music when they were young will continue to like this music for many years. Others will move on to other kinds of music. This gives a very mixed picture of musical tastes. But there are some music genres different age groups listen to. You can get an overview of the most popular genres in the Age-specific Music Genre Guide.

Age-specific Music Genre Guide

Age group Music Genre	20s	30s	40s	50s	60s
New Age		X	X	X	
Electronica		X	X		
Dance music	X	X			
House	X	X			
Hip-hop & Rap	X	X			
R 'n' B	X	X			
Soul		X	X	X	X
Blues			X	X	X
Pop	X	X	X		
Evergreens				X	X
Easy Listening			X	X	X
Latin Music	X	X	X	X	X
Classic Rock			X	X	X
Modern Rock	X	X	X		
Hard Rock & Metal	X	X			
Folk		X	X	X	X
Country	X	X	X	X	X
Jazz				X	X
Classical			X	X	X
Opera			X	X	X
Musicals			X	X	X

You do not have to become a lover or an expert of any music that you do not like in order to convey a youthful mind. It seems that many people have great difficulty in acknowledging music that they don't like. But being aware and acknowledging that there are types of music that certain age groups like—and which are different from your own personal taste—is a big step in communicating across generations. You can use the Age-specific Music Genre Guide to establish which music genres you like and find out if there are some other genres that are close to your taste—but more youthful—that may be worth getting to know better.

LITERARY STIMULATION FOR YOUTHFUL MINDS

A youthful mind is curious and open-minded. You can test whether this is the case for your mind with five books about youth and about being young.

F. Scott Fitzgerald:
This Side of Paradise
The book's back cover says it all: "Daring in intention, exuberant in execution, and audacious in its representation of the liberated American woman, *This Side of Paradise* is an uninhibited paean to American youth."

Muriel Spark:
The Prime of Miss Jean Brodie
"A perfect book" the *Chicago Tribune* called this book about a teacher in a staid girl's school in Edinburgh, Scotland. The cover is right when it claims that it's a dazzling psychological study, a darkly fascinating tale of treachery and passion.

J.D. Salinger:
Catcher in the Rye

The story of a couple of days in a sixteen-year-old boy's life just after he's been expelled from prep school; with his constant wry observations about what he encounters, from teachers to other phonies, the book captures the essence of the eternal teenage experience of alienation. One of the most important books to come out of the twentieth century.

Francesca Lia Block:
Weetzie Bat

This is what the *New York Times* said about this book: "*Weetzie Bat* burst on the young adult book scene like a rainbow bubble showering clouds of roses, feathers, tiny shells, and a rubber chicken. Hardened critics, who thought they'd seen all the possible variants of the coming-of-age novel, were astonished by the freshness of Francesca Lia Block."

Mark Salzman:
The Laughing Sutra

This is what *Washington Post Book World* wrote about this book: "A rich blend of fantasy, philosophy, history and romance. Salzman is a master storyteller and the fortunate reader will find himself entranced, entertained, and very definitely enlightened."

ENTERTAINMENT FOR
YOUTHFUL MINDS

Ten memorable movies about *being* young—in case you need to refresh your memory.

The Graduate
Graduating from college, and then what? Recent college graduate Benjamin Braddock starts an affair with Mrs. Robinson, the wife of his father's neighbor and business partner, and then finds himself falling in love with her teenage daughter, Elaine.

Roman Holiday
A young and innocent princess escapes from her "golden cage" and experiences life to the full in Rome with an American man. She doesn't know the man who befriends her is a reporter out for a story.

Almost Famous
William Miller is a fifteen-year-old boy, hired by *Rolling Stone* magazine to tour with, and write about, an up-and-coming rock band. This authentic coming-of-age film follows William as he falls face first while confronting life, love, and lingo.

Grease
Good girl Sandy and greaser Danny fell in love over the summer. After the summer holiday, they find out that they're now in the same high school, which causes conflicts and heartache for different people.

The Virgin Suicides
A group of male friends become obsessed with a group of beautiful sisters who are sheltered by their strict, religious parents after one of them commits suicide, but the sheltering ends up in more tragedy.

Romeo & Juliet

Shakespeare's famous play about two teenagers from rivaling families who meet, fall in love, and fight for their love despite their parents being enemies. There are different filmed versions of the tragedy.

Dead Poets' Society

Students at a boarding school meet Professor Keating, their new English teacher, who tells them of the Dead Poets Society, and encourages them to go against the status quo. Each, in his own way, does this, and is changed for life.

American Beauty

Parents and their children living under the same roof but having completely different lives. Daughter Jane is embarrassed about her parents while developing a happy friendship with a shy boy next door named Ricky who lives with a dominating father.

Forest Gump

Forrest Gump has both psychological and physical challenges in his young life, and he grows up experiencing the changes of the 1950s, 1960s, and 1970s, ending up accomplishing great things, including falling in love with a girl who does not feel the same way about him.

Donnie Darko

Teenager Donnie Darko tries to deal with people in his town, like the school bully, his conservative health teacher, and a self-help guru, while hearing the voice of an imaginary six-foot-tall bunny.

BE AWARE OF LIFE PHASES

How we look and the age we signal are important to many people. But looks are not the only key to well-being and feeling good about oneself. How we feel about our different life phases is equally important. This is why it is important to learn how to adjust to a new life phase.

Turning forty, fifty, or sixty years old represents not only biological changes, but also psychological changes. We may become aware that other people react to us in new ways, and we ourselves may observe changes in how we think and what is important to us. This is part of a natural process that most people experience. Of course, we may not be happy about it, and it can cause stress and depressive thoughts.

Growing older gives many people more insight into themselves, and some people become more confident and sure of themselves with age. But growing older also represents a loss or can be viewed as a loss—of youth, of good times, of health. We may not like it, but if we know how to say a proper "good bye" to the life phase that is over, we are likely to feel better about our next life phase. A proper good bye is quiet and invisible, and may take some time, maybe a couple of years or more.

People who are in denial of the changing life phases often get mental health problems because they do not acknowledge their loss, and thus they avoid the feelings associated with what they have lost.

Loss may be a dramatic word to use in this respect, but loss reflects that to some people it can be dramatic to turn fifty, sixty, or seventy and retire from the workplace and realize that there are fewer chances to do what you want to do in life.

Using the word loss also indicates that there can be a need for a grieving process when all these changes happen. Grieving is an unpleasant feeling, but when handled as a process of change, it can lead to new insights, new life skills, and a new outlook on life.

The more literally you can say good bye to what you have lost, the better chance you'll have of getting through the entire grieving process without mental health problems. This may involve stating one's loss to oneself, either by verbalizing it or writing about it. Sharing these thoughts with people who are or have been in the same situation can be beneficial—if they have adjusted well to their new life phase.

Grieving takes time. It may take weeks or months, but verbalizing the loss one is feeling to oneself and to close family and friends are the most important steps you can take to move on with your feelings.

On your way to looking younger

❖ How old you look is also influenced by your thinking.

❖ Stay tuned in to what goes on among people younger than yourself.

❖ Let music, books, and movies be an inspiration to stay youthful.

Getting Started

CHAPTER FOCUS

❖ Golden rules
❖ Planning
❖ People's comments

Now that you have an overview of how to look the age you feel rather than your biological age, it is time to get started on looking younger. You have to decide what will work best for you, and what you feel comfortable doing. Do you want to make just a few adjustments—or do you want a complete makeover? No matter what you decide, here is some helpful insight that will help get you started.

On television and in magazines, we can watch or read about people getting makeovers. Not all of these makeovers are about looking younger; many are about "dressing right" or dressing in a certain style. But there is no doubt that the makeovers that give the most striking results are the ones that do the most visually in the shortest time.

Now it is *your* turn to get a makeover! The best way of being successful at looking younger and getting the most striking results is also by following all the advice presented in this book in a relatively short time, say, a couple of months. It is probably only then you will get *Wow!* responses.

There may be several reasons why it may take longer than a couple of months, though. It costs money to buy new clothing, and you do not get a fitter body or lose weight in a short time. Also, maybe you do not feel the need to take all options mentioned in this book into account. You may choose to just use some of the information right now. At other times, you may want to use other parts.

But before starting on looking younger, let's have a look at what are NOT age revealers. Each of us has a beauty ideal, and in society, there are always certain prevalent beauty ideals. They will change from time to time, but they are visible everywhere we look. Looking younger in this book is not just about a certain beauty ideal. There are many elements in a person's appearance that have nothing to do with looking younger but are about a certain beauty ideal or about looking sexy.

What Are Not Age Revealers

The following elements in a person's appearance have nothing to do with looking younger. You have not found information on these issues in this book simply because they have no influence on looking younger. They are visual signals that are neutral age revealers. Having a gap between your teeth does not say anything about your age. Having a gap between her front teeth has never made singer Madonna, born in 1958, look older.

- ☑ Being pale
- ☑ Breast size
- ☑ Buttocks size
- ☑ Chin shape
- ☑ Ear size
- ☑ Eye color
- ☑ Feet size
- ☑ Gap between teeth
- ☑ Hair color
- ☑ Lip size
- ☑ Moles
- ☑ Nose size and shape
- ☑ Scars
- ☑ Skin problems

Many things about looks and beauty are not actually about age. If you are not happy about your appearance, this may affect how you approach life. Then you have to find out if you want to do something about what bothers you, what can be done, and plan what you want to do about it. Changing this will not automatically make you look younger, but you may end up looking more beautiful according to your own—and other peoples'—beauty ideals. It is important to be aware that you can look younger without changing what bothers you from a purely visual point of view because many of the things that may bother you could be age neutral.

This book presents many ways to look younger, but if we get to the core of it, there are Ten Golden Rules about looking younger. If you start by paying attention to these golden rules, you have a very good starting point.

The 10 Golden Rules of Looking Younger

The slimmer you are, the younger you look.

The fitter you are, the younger you look.

The more fashionably you dress, the younger you look.

The more fashionable accessories you wear, the younger you look.

The fewer wrinkles you have, the younger you look.

The whiter teeth you have, the younger you look.

The longer hair you have, the younger you look.

The less gray hair you have, the younger you look.

The less make-up you need to use, the younger you look.

The more fashionable the make-up you use, the younger you look.

Because not everything may be relevant, you need to make your own individual plan. You can do so by using this Easy-planner Checklist.

Easy-planner Checklist

1. First find out what you want to do.
2. Decide when you want to do it.
3. Do it.
4. Did it achieve what you expected?

Often, it will become more real if you write down what you want to do.

What I Want to Do	When I Want to Do It	Done or Not Done	How It Made Me Look and Feel

Your own comfort about the changes is the most important thing. Of course, it is always nice to get positive responses from other people. Some will volunteer their comments, but you have to prepare yourself that they may not always be positive. That does not mean that you have not achieved what *you* wanted and what this book is about. Actually, you may have achieved it too well. Some people do not like changes (even in other people), some will be envious of you because you look younger, some will feel that your efforts are unnecessary, or that you look ridiculous. There may be dozens of other explanations for negative comments. In order to find out how you should react to negative comments, try first to figure out the person's motive for saying what he or she does. While envy is unpleasant when we are confronted with it, it is a fact of life. When we are confronted with it, one way of dealing with it is accepting it as the other person's problem.

If you want to find out if you have succeeded in looking younger, ask people whom you trust to tell you their perceptions of you. This can be people that you already know—or it could be people that you have never met before or just barely know. When you start getting the same comments again and again, you are probably getting answers you can trust.

If you get comments that you can use, it is a good idea to keep track of them, especially if they make you feel good; they are worth remembering. You can use this log to keep track of comments.

Comments on My Look

Name	Comment	My Comments

Name	Comment	My Comments

On your way to looking younger

❖ Not everything in this book will work for you—
   focus on what will.

❖ Looking younger is not about adapting to all or
   certain beauty ideals—only the ones that make
   you look younger.

❖ Be prepared for both positive and negative
   comments about your youthful look.

❖ Consult the tools and guidelines in this book from
   time to time to see if something new has become
   relevant to you.

About the Author

Henrik Vejlgaard, M.Sc., M.A., is the author of three books on trends and lifestyle: *Anatomy of a Trend, The Lifestyle Puzzle*, and *Style Eruptions*. The books document how changes in style and taste take place, and how we communicate with the clothes we wear.

He coined the term "age-elasticity" in the late 1990s and became an expert in understanding the new concept of age, i.e., that there is a huge difference between biological age and self-perceived age.

He is also the author of *Look the Age You Feel: A Man's Guide to Looking Younger*, which is the men's version of *Look Younger Without Surgery*.

Other Books by Henrik Vejlgaard

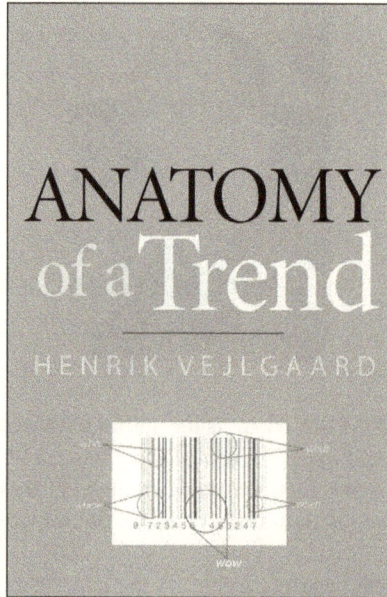

ANATOMY
of a Trend
HENRIK VEJLGAARD

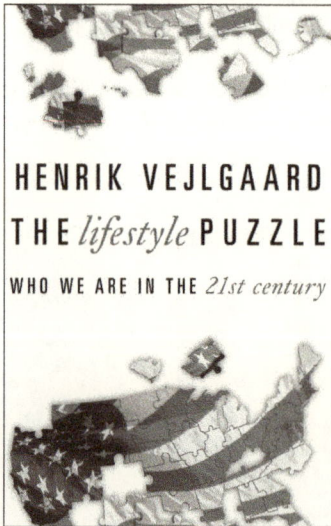

HENRIK VEJLGAARD
THE *lifestyle* PUZZLE
WHO WE ARE IN THE *21st century*

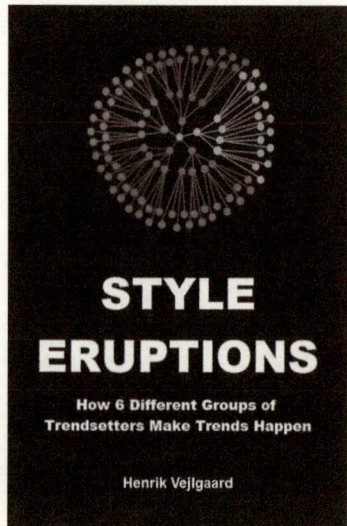

STYLE
ERUPTIONS

How 6 Different Groups of
Trendsetters Make Trends Happen

Henrik Vejlgaard

www.ingramcontent.com/pod-product-compliance
Lightning Source LLC
Chambersburg PA
CBHW030019290326
41934CB00005B/399